THE NUTRITION SUPERBOOK

2

# THE GOOD FATS AND OILS

KEATS TITLES OF RELATED INTEREST

*The Nutrition Superbook. Volume 1: The Antioxidants*
Jean Barilla, M.S.

*The Nutrition Desk Reference. 3rd Edition*
Robert H. Garrison, Jr., R.Ph. and Elizabeth Somer, M.A., R.D.

*Hypertension and Nutrition*
Eric R. Brayerman, M.D.

THE NUTRITION SUPERBOOK

2

# THE GOOD FATS AND OILS

EDITED BY

JEAN BARILLA, M.S.

KEATS PUBLISHING, INC.
NEW CANAAN, CONNECTICUT

The information contained in this book is not intended as medical advice. Its intention is solely informational and educational. Please consult a medical or health professional should the need for one be indicated.

THE NUTRITION SUPERBOOK: 2
THE GOOD FATS AND OILS



Library of Congress Cataloging-in-Publication Data
The Nutrition superbook / edited by Jean Barilla.
p. cm.
Includes bibliographical references and index.
Contents: v. 1. The antioxidants.
v. 2. The good fats and oils.
ISBN 0-87983-671-7 (vol. 1)
ISBN 0-87983-708-X (vol. 2)
1. Vitamins in human nutrition. 2. Antioxidants. I. Barilla, Jean.
QP771.N88 1995
612.3'99—dc20 95-11419
CIP

Printed in the United States of America

Published by Keats Publishing, Inc.
27 Pine Street, Box 876
New Canaan, Connecticut 06840-0876

10 9 8 7 6 5 4 3 2 1

*To*

people everywhere who want to
eat their fat and have it too.

# CONTENTS

A section of photographs appears after page 148

# PART ONE

# THE BASICS

# INTRODUCTION

EAT EGGS! Don't eat eggs! High cholesterol will kill you! Low cholesterol will kill you! High fat, low fat, no fat—what dietary fat level is best for you? The controversy rages and the battle continues. The food companies vie with each other to create products with less and the least fat. Corporate chemists create no-calorie fat substitutes with long-term health effects known only to those with functioning crystal balls. Who do we believe? What do we do?

*The Good Fats and Oils* will dispel the myths and give you the facts. Yes, there are fats and oils that are good for you! Many are essential for good health, even for life itself. This book will:

- Explain just what a fat is and what role fats play in the body.
- Introduce you to the key fats that you must get from your diet.
- Discuss the role of fats in disease.
- Reveal the studies that prove the benefits of certain fats and oils.
- Show you how to protect yourself from harmful effects of the fats you do eat.
- Provide information on the "fat partners"—substances that work with fats and oils to enhance their beneficial effects.

The fat and oily facts are right at your fingertips.

# KEY FATS AND RELATED MOLECULES

Before we can talk about good fats and oils, we have to know what these substances are. Fat is one of six groups of nutrients that are required for life and health, along with proteins, carbohydrates, vitamins, minerals and water. Fat is called "lipid" by biochemists. What we call "fat" is a lipid that is solid at room temperature; oil is a lipid that is liquid at that temperature.

Fats and oils are made up of building blocks called fatty acids. "Fatty" pertains to one end of the molecule that does not dissolve in water, while "acid" refers to the other end of the molecule that does dissolve in water. Fats and oils are also called triglycerides because they consist of three (*tri*) fatty acid molecules joined to a glycerol (a form of sugar) molecule. Lipids in the membranes that surround our cells are called phospholipids because the mineral phosphorus is part of the molecule.

## SATURATED WITH INFORMATION

Fatty acids are made up of atoms of carbon (C), hydrogen (H) and oxygen (O) linked together like chains.

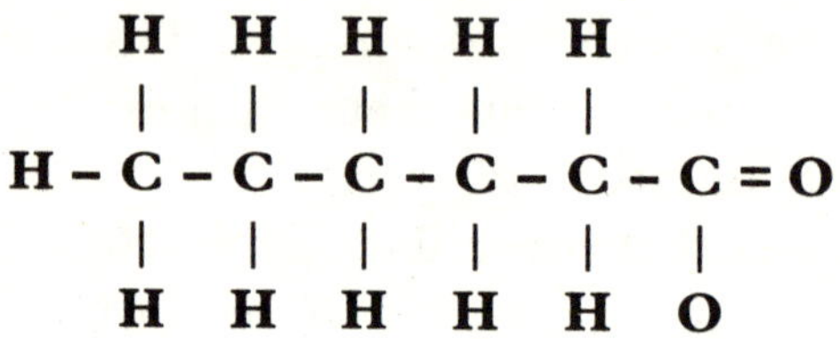

The lines between the atoms represent chemical bonds. One line indicates a single bond, two lines indicates a double bond.

When the chain of carbons has as many hydrogen atoms as it can possibly hold, and only has single bonds between the carbon atoms, the fat is called *saturated.* These fats are solid at room temperature. The greater the saturated fat content, the higher will be the melting temperature. Animal fats and two vegetable fats (oil from coconuts and palm kernels) are highly saturated. For most people, a diet high in saturated fat stimulates the liver to make so-called "bad" (low-density lipoprotein or LDL) cholesterol. The saturated molecules have a tendency to stick together. An excess can cause heart and blood vessel health problems.

When the chain has fewer hydrogen atoms, and double bonds between the carbons, the fat is *unsaturated* and will stay liquid in cold temperatures. Unsaturated fats tend to be anti-sticky and move apart, increasing fluidity. A monounsaturated fat has one carbon to carbon (C=C) double bond; examples are olive, canola, peanut and avocado oils. Polyunsaturated fats have two or more double bonds between carbons; examples are corn, soy, sesame, sunflower and safflower oils.

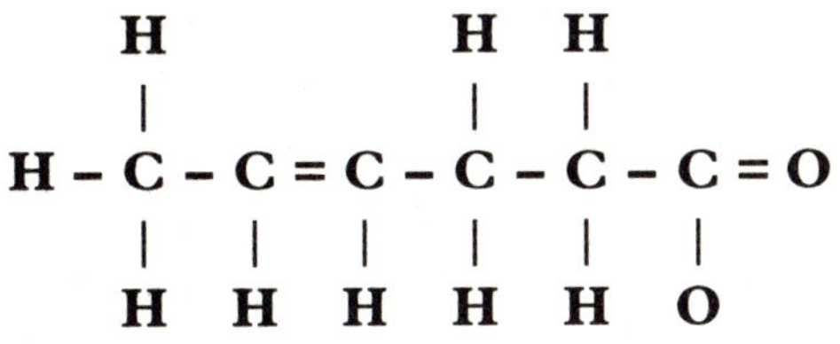

**MONOUNSATURATED**

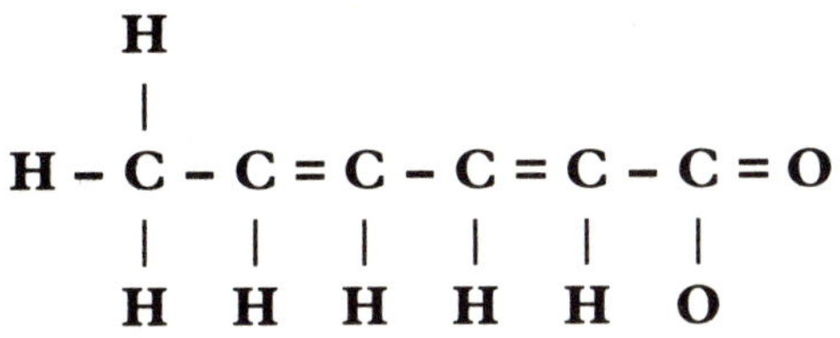

**POLYUNSATURATED**

To complicate things further, double bonds come in two types: *cis-* and *trans-*configurations. To understand what this terminology means, you first need to know that actual molecules are three-dimensional and bonds project in all directions from carbon atoms. An analogy would be a child's Tinker Toy set with the sticks (bonds) sticking out in all directions from the rounded connecting pieces (atoms). When both hydrogen atoms on the carbons involved in the double bond are on the same side of the molecule, the conformation is called cis. When the hydrogens are on opposite sides of the C=C bond, the conformation is called trans. The trans form makes the fat more stable (less likely to become rancid) than the cis form. Even though trans fats are unsaturated, they behave like saturated fats.

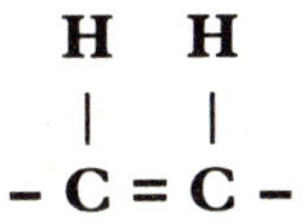

**CIS**

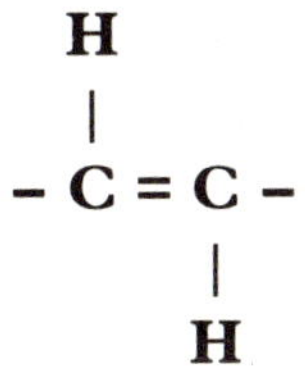

**TRANS**

The end of the fat molecule where three hydrogens are bonded to the carbon is called the methyl end. The numbering system for carbon atoms is the omega (w) system, where carbon atoms are numbered starting from the methyl end. Plant sources of fatty acids contain w-3 and w-6 forms, where the number indicates where the double bond is located. Fish oils also contain w-3 forms.

The essential fatty acids (EFAs), those that we cannot make and must obtain from foods, are linoleic acid (a w-6 form) and alpha-linolenic acid (a w-3 form).

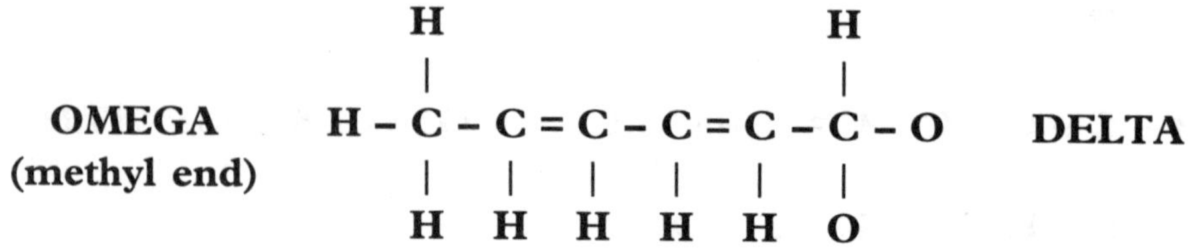


## FROM GOOD TO BAD

Hydrogenation is the most common way of changing healthful natural oils into products that can have major detrimental effects on our health. It is done by industry for one reason: to save money. Hydrogenated oils have a longer shelf life. Manufacturers can start with cheap, low-quality oils and turn them into margarines.

Hydrogenation (creating unnatural sources of saturated fat) adds hydrogen atoms in a chemical process that uses aluminum, a metal that may be linked to Alzheimer's disease (mental senility). If the fat is completely hydrogenated, where all double bonds in an oil are saturated with hydrogen, there are no cis or trans forms since there are no double bonds left. Hydrogenation also produces unnatural fatty acid fragments and other altered molecules, some of which may be toxic. The long-term effects of these substances are unknown. Hydrogenated fats include margarine, solid vegetable shortening and all processed foods made with partially hydrogenated oils.

Partial hydrogenation, leaving some double bonds, results in fats that have both cis and trans molecules. Trans fatty acids interfere with body biochemistry. While the body can make cell membranes and hormones from cis fatty acids, it is not known what is done with the trans forms. Trans fatty acids have been shown to increase cholesterol levels, decrease the "good" (high-density lipoprotein or HDL) cholesterol, interfere with the detoxification system in the liver and affect essential fatty acid metabolism.

## THE IMPORTANCE OF FATS AND OILS IN BODY STRUCTURE AND FUNCTION

Fats and oils provide or are important structural and functional components in our bodies. Without them we could not survive.

### WHAT FATS DO

1. Provide energy for physical processes, i.e., muscle function, breathing, growth and repair.
2. Serve as padding or insulation around vital body organs and act as a shock absorber to protect the organs from injury during average physical exertion and movement.
3. Help conserve body heat by providing warmth from within the body.
4. Transport vitamins such as A, D, E. and K (the "fat soluble" vitamins) through the blood.
5. Act as an intestinal lubricant to facilitate elimination.
6. Build body cells by combining with the mineral phosphorus (as phospholipids) to form cell walls.
7. Act as insulation for nerves, i.e., the myelin sheath.
8. Provide essential fatty acids (arachidonic, linoleic and linolenic) that promote growth of cells, tissues and organs.
9. Make foods more palatable and enjoyable, helping you feel fuller and more satisfied for a longer period of time than other food classes.

Essential fatty acids (linoleic and linolenic) are necessary for energy production, utilization of oxygen, production of red blood pigment (hemoglobin) and are part of the cell membranes that allow nutrients in and wastes out of our cells. These fats help our muscles recover from fatigue and are used to make prostaglandins—the hormone-like substances that regulate blood pressure, among other things. Essential fatty acids are also important in cell growth and division, in keeping the skin smooth, in promoting healing and for brain development in children.

Triglycerides are the main type of fats that we eat and store as body fat. Although an overabundance of these fats in the bloodstream can increase the risk of heart disease, they are also important for body metabolism. Note that triglycerides cause trouble when they oxidize and damage blood vessel linings. Antioxidant nutrients such as vitamins C and E, carotenes, selenium, zinc and manganese help prevent such oxidation. For a detailed discussion of antioxidant nutrients, see Volume 1 of this Nutrition Superbook series, *The Antioxidants*.

Triglycerides help insulate our bodies from the cold by forming a fat layer just under our skin. These fats act as a shock absorber for internal organs and other body structures. The main function of triglycerides is as a storage form of energy that can be used when needed.

Phospholipids, which are similar to triglycerides in structure, are essential components of the membranes that surround our cells and the fats that float in our bloodstream. They form a barrier around cells, allowing entry and exit of substances necessary for cell function. One dietary phospholipid, lecithin, can help keep cholesterol from damaging arteries and prevent and dissolve gall and kidney stones. Choline, a B vitamin, is used to make lecithin and also the neurotransmitter acetylcholine. Inositol, another B vitamin, stimulates proper management of fats in the liver. These "fat partners" will be discussed in Part III of this book.

Cholesterol can be detrimental to our health, but we could not survive without it. Along with phospholipids, it is an integral part of the cell membrane, a regulator of the consistency of the membrane. Cholesterol is also the material from which our body makes steroid hormones such as estrogen, testosterone and the adrenal hormones that regulate blood pressure and decrease inflammation. Cholesterol is also used to make bile acids, to digest and absorb fats in our diet, and to protect our skin from dryness.

## FAT METABOLISM

Fats, as noted above, are made of glycerol and saturated, monounsaturated and essential fatty acids. Glycerol can be used to make glucose when we run low on this sugar. Saturated fatty acids are mainly used as fuel that our body "burns" to produce energy. When we take in too many calories, our body stores the excess as fat to prevent the metabolic "fire" from getting too hot.

Monounsaturated fatty acids can also be used to produce energy. When the body is low in essential fatty acids, the monounsaturated fats can be converted and partially serve the function of these essential fats. We only burn essential fatty acids for energy when there is an excess. They are better used to make phospholipids for the cell membranes and take part in many vital biological processes.

There are other substances that act as fat partners and help the body metabolize fats and are of value as nutrients themselves (see Part III). Octacosanol, isolated from wheat germ oil, can improve muscle endurance and lower cholesterol levels. Both race horses and human athletes have realized improved performance from this good oil.

Carnitine is an amino acid (a building block of proteins) that is responsible for the body's ability to metabolize fat for energy. It can also lower elevated triglyceride levels, thus decreasing the risk of blood vessel disease. We can make carnitine in our bodies, but only if we have other key nutrients available to do so.

Taurine, another amino acid, works with bile acids in the liver to keep cholesterol soluble, thus preventing gallstones. We can make it, but only in limited amounts. It is important for the health of the heart, eyes and nervous system. Women may have a greater need for this nutrient.

Sesame seed, besides being an excellent source of highly unsaturated fatty acids, contains two important amino acids. Methionine, crucial for keeping the liver healthy, also is converted to choline when there is an excess of it. Choline, as mentioned above, helps handle cholesterol and helps the body produce energy. The other amino acid, tryptophan, can provide the B vitamin niacin which lowers cholesterol. Sunflower and pumpkin seeds are also excellent sources of nutrients as are wheat and corn germs.

Lipoic acid is called the metabolic antioxidant. It is a unique nutrient that is part of a network that protects the fats that are part of cell membranes from becoming rancid. It also helps convert food fats into energy. One of the most important functions of lipoic acid is to help prevent LDL cholesterol from becoming a menace to our blood circulatory system.

You are invited to open the pages of this book and learn, in depth, the facts about fats that will help you live a longer, healthier and happier life.

# PART TWO

# THE OILS WE NEED

# EPA—MARINE LIPIDS

*In the Battle Against Heart Disease—An Answer Comes from the Sea*

RICHARD A. PASSWATER, PH.D.

A FOIL FOR HEART TROUBLE

Why don't the Eskimos and the Japanese succumb to coronary attacks like the rest of us? The reason is, according to the researchers and numerous successful clinical studies, because they eat mostly cold salt-water, fatty fish such as cod, mackerel and herring. Fatty fish supply EPA (eicosapentaenoic acid) which can control blood clotting, artery spasms, cholesterol and triglycerides, the vital factors in ailing hearts. This is the story of EPA and the marine lipids, our surprising insurance against cardiovascular trouble.

## COLD-WATER FISH OILS—EPA AND DHA

Nutritional research revealed over a decade ago important evidence that a concentration of certain marine lipids in the blood protects against heart disease, improves gland and enzyme function, and plays a vital role in brain and nerve health.

The wide involvement of fish oils from cold-water fish in so many basic areas of health finds its source in two main nutrients. One influences prostaglandin (hormone-like compounds) balance and the other is needed by brain and nerve cells. Yet both of these nutrients are now sparse in modern Western diets. As they have disappeared from our diets, the incidence of heart disease has increased.

The nutrient receiving the widest interest is EPA (eicosapentaenoic acid) which is required for the production of the prostaglandin-3 family that controls blood clotting and artery spasms. EPA also improves blood viscosity, lowers cholesterol (especially the cholesterol bound to low-density lipoprotein which is believed to be a risk factor in heart disease), and lowers triglycerides.

Of almost equal importance, but as yet not as widely researched is DHA (docosahexaenoic acid), although it comes from the same source as EPA. DHA is a major component of the brain and retina, and has a possible role in nerve transmission.

Both of these nutrients belong to a special class of highly concentrated, long-chained, polyunsaturated fatty acids that biochemists call "omega-3" fatty acids. They differ markedly from the common fatty acids found in vegetables which are mostly "omega-6" fatty acids and are really di-unsaturated, rather than polyunsaturated. (This distinction and its importance will be made clear later.)

For many decades, researchers have been trying to solve the mystery of heart disease in terms of cholesterol and fats. It has been animal fats against vegetable fats, even though animal fats contain some polyunsaturated fats and vegetables contain some saturated fats. The Eskimo poses the enigma—the Eskimo who consumes a native diet rich in animal fat yet is virtually free of the heart disease that is the major killer of Americans and Europeans. The Japanese also suffer fewer coronaries than Easterners. The one factor common to both the Eskimo and Japanese that is lacking in the Westerner's diet involves the amount of cold salt-water fatty fish consumed.

The link between the consumption of deep sea fish and the reduced incidence of heart disease was responsible for research that upset a previous concept. The concept that the ratio of polyunsaturated fat to saturated fat is important turns out to be not only the wrong approach but possibly a harmful approach. This approach can discourage us from taking correct action and it can also unbalance our diet further so as to increase the incidence of several diseases, including cancer.

Research has showed scientists that they should be improving the omega-3 balance to omega-6 and omega-9 fats. This chapter hopes to point out why a balance of fatty acids is just as important to health as is a balance of amino acids, vitamins and minerals.

When herring, cod and mackerel are abundantly added to Western diets, blood changes occur that mimic the protective changes in the blood of the Eskimo. Since most North Americans and Europeans easily tire of daily rations of fatty fish, extracts were prepared to see if the same beneficial results could be achieved. The specially selected marine lipids concentrated in the extract called MaxEPA*™ produced the beneficial results; thus MaxEPA is being used extensively by medical researchers.

This line of research was conducted at prestigious universities and clinics in the United States and Europe and supported by organizations such as the American Heart Association, the National Institutes of Health, the Danish Heart Association, British Cancer Campaign, Danish Foundation for Medical Research, and others.

The results have been reported throughout the medical establishment and in general news magazines for many years.

The January 18, 1982 *Medical World News* reports, "Fish-oil diet said to reduce lipids (cholesterol and triglycerides) sharply. A salmon a day may keep a coronary away." The article reported on the research of Dr. William Connor, Professor of Medicine and then head of the clinical nutrition section and lipid atherosclerosis laboratory at the Oregon Health Sciences University in Portland. He found that fish oil lowered blood cholesterol, triglycerides, low-density lipoproteins (LDL), and raised the beneficial high-density lipoproteins (HDL), improving the clotting factors.

The information was also reported in an article entitled, "It's Not Fishy: Fruit of the Sea May Foil Cardiovascular Disease," in the February 12, 1982 issue of the *Journal of the American Medical Association.*

*™Seven Seas Health Care Ltd., Hull, England. North America: R. P. Scherer Corp.

Newspapers carried the following quote attributed to Dr. Connor by United Press International: "I think we have new hope for preventing the development of coronary heart disease with rather simple dietary modifications."

The February 9, 1981 *U.S. News & World Report* discussed how "a key fatty acid, EPA, dramatically inhibits formation of blood clots." The article quotes Dr. Philip Needleman, head of the department of pharmacology at Washington University Medical School in St. Louis, as saying ". . . we might think about taking a capsule of enriched oil from this fish."

EPA research was mentioned in *Family Circle* (January 12, 1982) as a means of reducing the painful inflammation of rheumatoid arthritis, as well as combating heart disease.

This early EPA research was obviously very exciting. Many studies have since confirmed the results mentioned above and have shown additional health benefits of EPA and DHA.

The high incidence of cardiovascular disease and mortality is not exclusively an American problem. It exists in industrialized nations around the world.

It is little wonder, therefore, that scientists, researchers and physicians in this country and abroad have been waging a battle against heart disease. In their search for an answer to this killer, experts have found an important clue to understanding the metabolism of the human body. The clue was found in, of all places, the sea.

During the 1970s, epidemiological studies of Eskimos and Japanese living by the sea were conducted. The studies showed that both populations had a relatively low incidence of coronary heart disease. The life expectancy of the Japanese over the age of twenty-five exceeded that of Americans. The life expectancy of Eskimos is not as good as that of Americans, but heart disease is rare even in the oldest Eskimos.

The Japanese diet has often been compared to the American diet. Increased amounts of vegetables, fish and the mineral selenium have been noted in the Japanese diet, but the Eskimo diet has fewer vegetables, less fiber and more fat and cholesterol. Both Japanese and Eskimo populations have diets which include substantial amounts of fatty fish, fish oil and other marine life.[1,2,3] (The selenium content of the Eskimo diet has not been studied, but fish are excellent sources of selenium.)

## WHAT ARE FATTY ACIDS?

In order to understand the link between fish diets and the lower rate of heart disease, it is necessary to explain some basic chemistry about the human body's metabolism—and this involves a description of fatty acids.

Fatty acids can be described as the chemical building blocks from which fats and oils (which chemists call "lipids") are made. They are composed of chains of molecules which, for the purpose of clarity, may be thought of as necklaces. There are short chains and longer chains. All of them are strung together with carbon atoms. When the chain contains hydrogen on any open links along with the carbon atoms, the result is a saturated fat. (See Figure 1A.) Most saturated fats come from animal sources such as beef fat, pork fat and butterfat.

Other fats and oils are described as being unsaturated. In this case, the carbon atoms instead of being connected to hydrogen atoms, turn back and connect to each other. The connection is called a double link or a double bond. (See Figure 1B arrow)

When the carbon atoms of the fatty acid are connected to each other with only one double link and no hydrogen, the fatty acid is termed "unsaturated."

When there are two double links and no hydrogen, they are called "di-unsaturated." (See Figure 1C.)

And, when there are more than two double links and no hydrogen, the correct terminology is "polyunsaturated."

Unsaturated or polyunsaturated fats are usually derived from vegetable or from marine sources, such as olive oil, sunflower seed oil, or cod liver oil. (Examples are given in Appendix A.)

FIGURE 1

FATTY ACID SATURATION

A

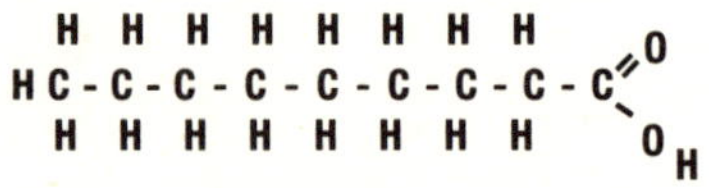

**Saturated**

B

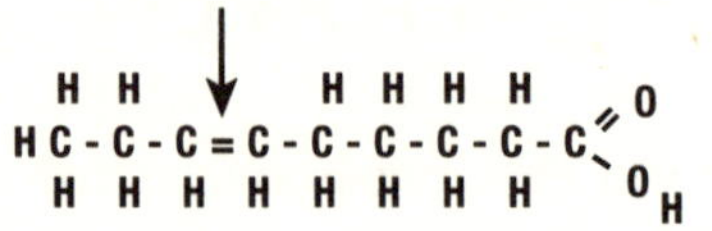

**Monounsaturated**

C

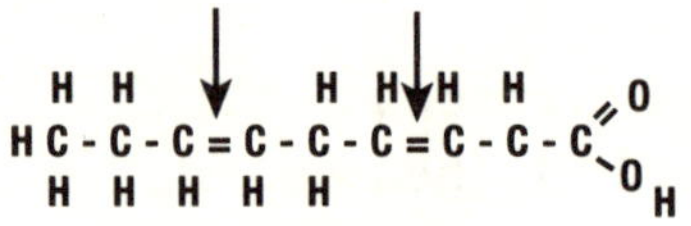

**Polyunsaturated**
**(PUFA)**
**(actually a di-unsaturated in this example)**

Most vegetable and seed oils are medium-sized chains while butterfats are shorter chains. Fish or other marine oils are unique because they are relatively long chains with many links. These long-chained fatty acids give to fish and other marine life the characteristic "fishy" odor and flavor.

The number of double links can also be used for identification. When there are 18 carbon atoms strung together without hydrogen and with one double link, the result is oleic acid; with two double links, the result is linoleic acid; with three double links, the result is linolenic acid. The last is a common component of linseed oil.

Dietary fatty acids are used within the body for a variety of purposes. They are needed to improve the health of the body, enter into the process of metabolism, maintain better function of the organs, and to keep the bloodstream healthy. If dietary fatty acids are not suitable for use, they can be converted to a degree, into the required kind, although this ability varies from species to species. Man appears to be able to increase the length of the carbon chain and to add double links in certain positions, but without dependable efficiency.

Another method of identification is called "numbering." If you imagine opening the clasp on the chain and laying the necklace on a table, the carbon atoms would be arranged from left to right. We could call the first carbon atom number 1, the second number 2, and so on. When the double link starts on the third carbon, the fatty acid is called omega-3 (w-3 or n-3) fatty acids.

When the double link starts on the sixth carbon, the fatty acid is referred to as omega-6 (w-6 or n-6) fatty acids.

Although man can convert some small chains to larger chains, the position of the double link remains the same so omega-3 cannot be converted to omega-6 under any circumstances. (See Figure 2.)

FIGURE 2

DIAGRAMMATIC REPRESENTATION OF THE FATTY ACIDS

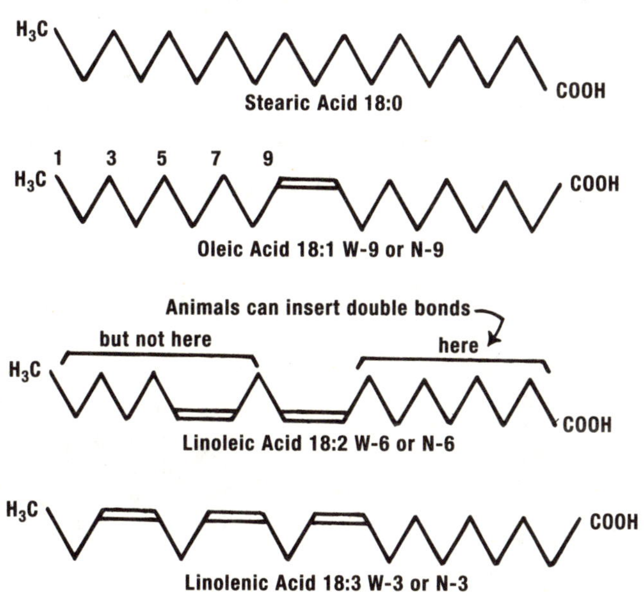

## ISOMERS

Compounds with the same atoms arranged in different order are called isomers. Some arrangements are called "cis" and others are called "trans."

Although they have the same basic structure, they are not interchangeable in cells. Trans-structures resemble the saturated oils, while cis-structures appear entirely different with sort of a horseshoe shape. (See Figure 3.) This shape occupies considerably more space than the same atoms arranged in a straight line—a small, but important difference.

Vegetable oils contain generous amounts of the cis-polyunsaturated fatty acids. However, commercial processing to improve stability and odor converts a substantial amount of the cis-polyunsaturated fatty acids to the trans-shape. Also, when vegetable or seed oils are hydrogenated (hydrogen atoms are added to the chain), to improve consistency and stability as in the production of margarine, not only are saturated fats formed but trans-shape fatty acids as well. For example:

- Stick margarine contains from 25 to 35 percent trans-fatty acids.
- Tub margarine contains from 15 to 25 percent trans-fatty acids.
- Shortening contains from 20 to 30 percent trans-fatty acids.
- Salad oils from 0 to 15 percent trans-fatty acids.

FIGURE 3

ISOMERS: THE SAME ATOMS, DIFFERENT ORDERS

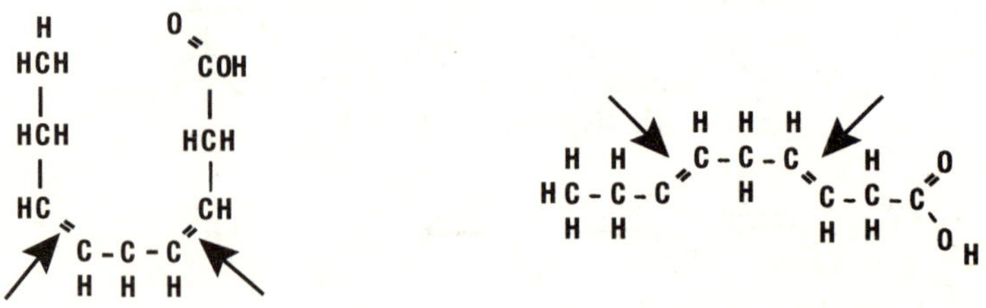

CIS TRANS

Trans-fatty acids have different chemical reactions than cis-fatty acids. They increase the fatty acid requirements and aggravate the symptoms of fatty acid deficiency. Trans-fatty acids are incorporated differently into cell membranes, thus affecting their function. They are also incorporated differently into triglycerides and phospholipids. An even more important characteristic is that trans-fatty acids greatly affect the utilization of fatty acids.

So, the characteristics of each fatty acid include:

the length of the chain
the number of double links
the location of the double links
whether the fatty acid is "cis" or "trans"

Table 1 compares the characteristics of several fatty acids.

TABLE 1 IMPORTANT DIETARY FATTY ACIDS

| Name | Carbon Atoms | Saturation |
|---|---|---|
| Stearic Acid | (18) | (Saturated) |
| Oleic Acid | (18:1;9) | (Monounsaturated) |
| Linoleic Acid | (18:2;9,12) | (W-6) |
| Alpha-Linolenic Acid | (18:3;9,12,15) | (W-3) |
| Gamma-Linolenic Acid | (18:3;6,9,12) | (W-6) |
| Arachidonic Acid | (20:4;5,8,11,14) | (W-6) |
| Eicosapentaenoic Acid | (20:5;5,8,11,14,17) | (W-3) |

## THE POTENT PROSTAGLANDINS

Once fat is converted into fatty acids, the body continues its metabolic processes, either burning them for energy, storing them for later use, or synthesizing the acids into what are termed prostaglandins (PGs)

Prostaglandins were discovered in the 1970s and research to date has shown that they affect diverse and potent biologic activities, behaving much like hormones.[4,5]

When the chemistry of the PGs was first unravelled, fatty acids having 20 carbon atoms (long chain) began to take on new significance. This was because of the discovery that PGs were 20 carbon molecules produced by partial oxidation of 20 carbon fatty acids. Long-chain polyunsaturates unique to fish oil, and in particular to EPA, were thus seen as precursors of PGs and the realization of their potential significance began to dawn.

The reason that we need the body well-stocked with the proper fatty acids is so that it can make as much prostaglandin as it needs. (See Figure 4.) The various human PGs are not readily obtainable in the diet, and if they were, since they are complex molecules, they would mostly be destroyed by the digestive process. Therefore, we should fortify our body's own production of PGs to assure an optimal supply.

*Why?* Because PGs control a multitude of essential functions in the body in relation to such seemingly unrelated disorders as heart attacks, high blood pressure, arthritis, menstrual cramps, allergies, asthma, migraine headaches, fertility, glaucoma and, perhaps, cancer.

Because PGs are not stored, every tissue makes them as needed. Their effect is brief since they are quickly inactivated by enzymes. Some organ systems depend on a balance of PGs which act in opposite ways.

In recent years scientists have learned of the functions of approximately twenty different PGs. Of them, the families designated as E family and F family are the most important. They are abbreviated for convenience as PGE and PGF. One other PG family is of particular interest, that of the "I" family. One member of the PGI family, $PGI_2$, often called "prostacyclin," is a particularly potent cellular regulator and anti-clotting agent. The most interesting family, however, is PGE and the most interesting members of this family are $PGE_1$ and $PGE_3$.

The subscripts refer to the fatty acids used as the starting point in production. The prostaglandin series made from gamma linolenic

FIGURE 4

CONVERSION OF LINOLENIC ACID TO PROSTAGLANDINS

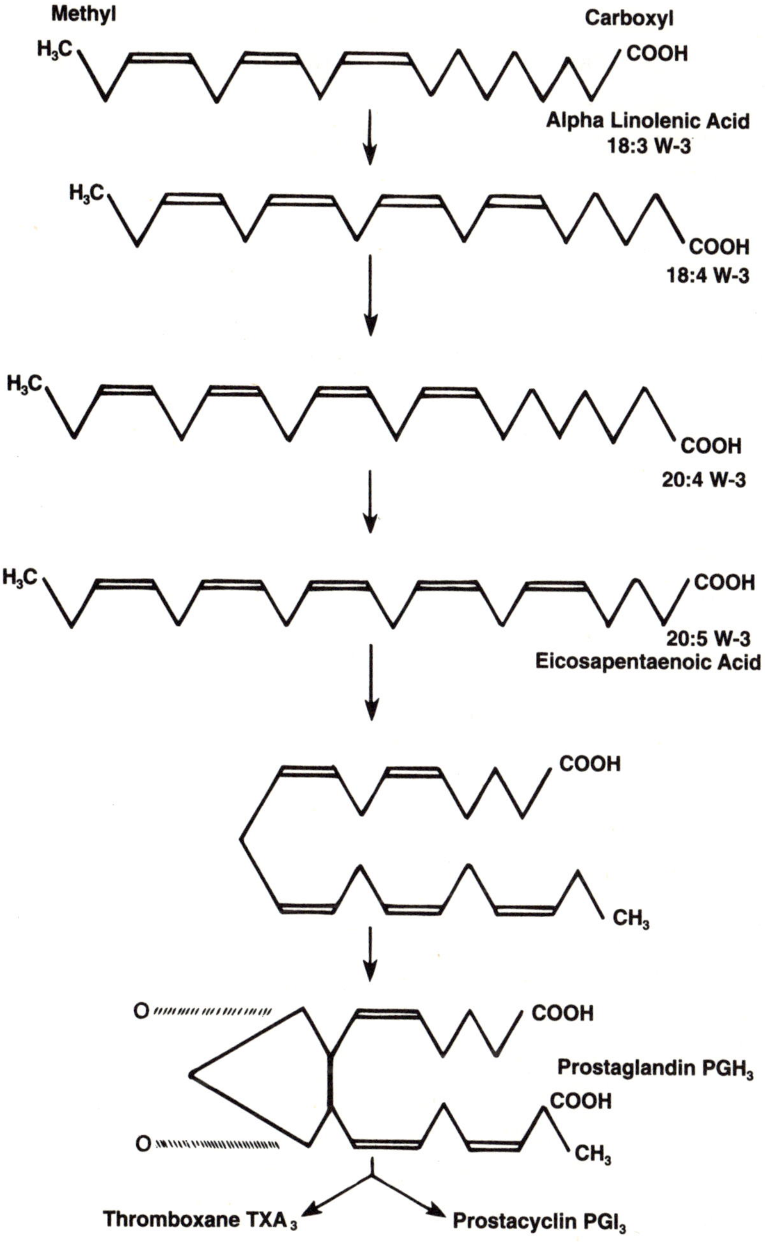

acid is designated by the subscript 1. The series made from arachidonic acid (AA) is designated by the subscript 2, and the series from eicosapentaenoic acid (EPA) by the subscript 3. The biological differences between the three series seem to depend solely on the differences in the number and position of the double links in the starting point—the particular fatty acid.

One well-acknowledged role of PGs is their involvement with blood clotting.

## BLOOD CLOTTING

Blood clotting is controlled by components in the blood called "platelets." Platelets are less than half the size of red blood cells and are shaped like plates. There are about 200,000 platelets in a cubic millimeter of blood. Platelets initiate blood clotting by forming a "clump" to which fibrin (a protein that assists the clotting of blood) can adhere. Platelets group together or aggregate around breaks or leaks in the blood vessels to prevent serious loss of blood.

The tendency of platelets to adhere to each other can be measured in the laboratory by determining the percentage of platelets that will stick to glass beads when the platelets are passed over the glass beads. This measurement is called the platelet adhesion index.

In 1972, a series of reports from Sweden noted that patients who had recovered from heart attacks had a shorter blood clotting time (stickier blood) than a population sample of the same age and sex.[6]

Normal blood has a platelet adhesion index of 20 to 35. Persons who have just experienced a heart attack have platelet adhesion indices over 90 and coronary-prone individuals have indices of 50 or greater.

Prostaglandins and prostaglandin derivatives affect blood clotting by either promoting or inhibiting this aggregation of platelets. The determination as to whether a PG is pro-aggregatory or anti-aggregatory is believed to be determined by the fatty acid from which the prostaglandin originates. Platelets can also adhere to injuries on the interior surface (endothelium) of the blood vessels and around abnormal cells growing in the arteries. The danger is that in some cases the platelets continue to congregate and form clots that block blood flow.

When this occurs in a coronary artery leading to the heart, the clot (thrombosis) can lead to heart damage (myocardial infarction). Blocking an artery that supplies blood to the brain can cause a stroke. Even a clot which forms in an arm or leg blood vessel can be extremely serious since it can block blood flow to the limb, or the clot can break off from its original site and be carried in the bloodstream until it lodges in another part of the body.

## CHOLESTEROL AND TRIGLYCERIDES

Blood platelet aggregation can also promote plaque build-up in the artery walls. The plaque contains fibrous materials, cholesterol, and other substances.

Cholesterol does not initiate this process but is involved in formation of the plaque. Research has indicated that platelet adhesion is very important and that the role of dietary cholesterol is not as crucial as once believed. Cholesterol exists in all animal tissue and has important biochemical properties for animals. Scientists can now detect five different kinds of cholesterol in the blood. One type of cholesterol—low-density lipoprotein or LDL cholesterol—is hazardous when damaged and has a greater likelihood of building up along artery walls. Another form of cholesterol—high-density lipoprotein or HDL cholesterol—is beneficial and may play a role in removing unwanted types of cholesterol from the body.[7,8,9]

Another factor that some consider in the relation between diet and heart disease is a class of compounds called triglycerides. A triglyceride consists of a molecule of glycerol that has three molecules of fatty acids attached. Glycerol itself is a 3-carbon atom chain having an alcohol (hydroxyl) group of atoms attached to each carbon atom.

Dietary fats are normally triglycerides. During digestion, the triglycerides are broken down by pancreatic lipase (steapsin) into mostly glycerol and free fatty acids. However, some diglycerides and monoglycerides remain as a result of incomplete digestion. The free fatty acids, glycerol, monoglycerides and diglycerides are absorbed with the aid of bile salts. The fatty materials are then reformed into triglycerides which circulate in the blood.

High levels of triglycerides in the blood are believed to be associated with an increased risk of heart disease.

## SIGNIFICANCE OF EPIDEMIOLOGICAL STUDIES

Now let's go back to the studies of the Eskimos and the Japanese living near the sea.

The diet of both of these populations was very high in fatty fish, fish oil, and other marine life. These people were found to have low levels of triglycerides, high levels of "good" HDL cholesterol, and a relatively reduced tendency for their blood to clot. And, as would be expected from these serum levels, both populations had a very low incidence of coronary heart disease.

Further study showed that these people had high levels of particular fatty acids, namely eicosapentaenoic acid (EPA) and docosahexaenoic acid (DHA) in their blood.[10]

Apparently EPA and DHA originate far down the food chain in minute free-floating plants and animals in the ocean which serve as direct or indirect food sources for all sea creatures. The acids are only found in significant quantities in fish, fish oils, and the fat of marine mammals who live on fish. Of course, these were the mainstay of the diet of the populations being studied.

EPA and DHA are not found in significant amounts in vegetable oils, land animals, or dairy products. The author suspects, however, that animal brains would be shown to contain significant amounts of DHA.

Both EPA and DHA are long chain, omega-3 fatty acids. EPA has a 20-carbon chain with five double links and DHA has a 22-carbon chain with six double links. It is interesting to note that it was not until the early 1970s that scientists paid much attention to fatty acids such as these which were more than 18 carbons long.

In examining the implications of EPA and DHA in the human diet, researchers reflected on historical changes in the eating habits of Western society. Their investigation proved that over the past 100 years, the amount of fatty fish consumed and the related intake of EPA and DHA has dropped significantly.[11] They attributed this change largely to the public's preference for non-oily fish which became more readily available through the advent of modern transportation and also because of the increase in the price of fish relative to other forms of protein.

The American diet, as well as the diets of other nations, changed to include higher amounts of animal meat, vegetable oils and other saturated fats. The diet became almost devoid of EPA and DHA. At the same time, cardiovascular disease escalated.

Only a few isolated populations continued to consume a diet rich in fatty fish—such as the Eskimos and the Japanese living by the sea. What further information could researchers gain from these populations about the relevance of their diet and protection from heart problems?

In order to properly assess the significance of a diet rich in fatty fish, a comparative study was made of fishing communities and farming communities in Japan. The study showed that the fishing communities had a higher daily intake of fish than the farming communities and correspondingly, the fishermen had significantly higher levels of EPA and DHA in their blood. The fishermen also had a reduced tendency towards blood platelet aggregation.[12]

Based on the results of this and other studies, researchers concluded that a diet which includes large amounts of fatty fish may increase the levels of EPA and DHA in the blood and this, in turn, might help avoid cardiovascular problems.

A new question then arose: Was there a need to supplement the diet of Western populations with foods rich in EPA and DHA, and if so, what effect would this have? In accordance with accepted scientific practice, these questions would be examined through research and experiments.

Sen et al.[13] fed sardine oil to rats which were stressed by being fed cholesterol and bile salt. The test diets incorporated not only hydrogenated vegetable oil, but also varying amounts of sardine oil, either from crude or processed oil or in the form of whole sardine fish.

The diets were adjusted so that the lipids contributed by the sardine oil were about 5 percent of the diet and overall lipid content was about 13 percent. The test ran about two months. It was found that the rats fed on either sardine oil or whole sardines had significantly lower levels of serum cholesterol.

Ruiter et al. fed groups of six young pigs on either mackerel oil supplemented diets or olive oil supplemented diets.[14] The oil supplement was given at the rate of 8 to 10 percent by weight of the diet. The animals were kept on the diet for four weeks. They observed lower levels of blood glucose and triglycerides and lower hemoglobin levels. They also concluded that one of the animals of the six involved showed symptoms of yellow fat disease and that four of the six treated with fish oil showed lipofuscin pigment development. These are both symptoms of selenium and/or vitamin E deficiency and calculation of the vitamin E and selenium intakes suggests that this was possible. Hornstra also found signs of yellow fat disease in rats fed cod liver oil and both these papers underline the well-established fact that extra dietary polyunsaturates must be accompanied by supplementary vitamin E to counteract the increased potential for oxidation of these highly labile materials.[15]

Hornstra showed that the rats fed cod liver oil had a reduced clotting tendency as well as reduced levels of $PGI_2$ and $TXA_2$. In a further paper, Hornstra confirmed the anti-clotting properties of cod liver oil, suggesting that because of the lack of evidence of enhanced $PGI_3$ production, the effect must have been due to an intrinsic plasma anti-clotting factor present in cod liver oil.[16]

Researchers around the world had conducted experiments to explore the significance and safety of an EPA and DHA-rich diet. The results of these studies conclusively showed that animals fed EPA and DHA-rich foods and oils had lower levels of "bad" or LDL cholesterol, a reduced blood clotting tendency, and, in general, better protection from cardiovascular disease than a control group. And these experiments clearly demonstrated the safety of a diet rich in EPA and DHA.

## HUMAN CLINICAL STUDIES

One of the first human studies reported was conducted by Von Lossonczy et al. in 1978.[17] He used Cistercian monks and nuns in a three-week, cross-over design experiment in which they were given a daily portion of mackerel which is rich in EPA and DHA. During the low omega-3 fatty acid period, cheese was substituted for the mackerel.

During the initial EPA-rich diet period, the volunteers' serum cholesterol and triglyceride levels dropped, but after three weeks on the cheese, these levels had been restored.

Van Gent et al. fed groups of ten nonfish-eating volunteers a fish oil concentrate containing 81 percent omega-3 acids including 25 percent EPA and 38 percent DHA.[18] They found that at intakes of up to 8 grams per day of omega-3 fatty acids for four weeks, there was no significant change in serum cholesterol or HDL cholesterol. Serum triglycerides and VLDL (very low denisty lipoprotein) did, however, fall significantly. The lack of effect on HDL cholesterol may have been due to the possibility that they used an omega-3 supplement based on ethyl esters. Such a form of presentation has been known to show different effects from that given by an omega-3-EPA.[19]

Mackerel was also used in a study by Siess et al.[20] These workers fed volunteers for a week on a diet containing 500 to 800 grams of stewed or smoked mackerel, together with a source of carbohydrate (unspecified). They found a marked decrease in the clumping and unwanted stickiness of blood platelets.

Harris and Conner[21] fed salmon oil diets to volunteers for four weeks. The diets were formulated to provide almost half of the calories as fat. On the treatment diet, the fat was omega-3 fatty acids while the control diet contained no omega-3 fatty acids. They found that after four weeks on the salmon meat/salmon oil diet, their subjects showed significantly lower levels of total cholesterol, serum triglycerides, VLDL cholesterol, and LDL cholesterol. HDL cholesterol was not significantly altered. It was also observed that clearance of serum triglycerides after a 50-gram fat load was also much faster when the fat was salmon oil rather than a control fat. The author also reported prolonged clotting time and reduced platelet counts.

Dyerberg et al.[22] showed that cod liver oil produced a change in plasma lipid after one week, while linseed oil in comparable quantities had much less effect. This suggests that man has a limited capacity to convert long chain fatty acids to longer chains and that dietary linoleic acid in linseed oil is not an effective means of providing EPA.

Sanders and Younger[23] studied the influence of one milliliter linseed oil supplement a day for two weeks on platelet and plasma lipids in four vegans (people who eat foods of plant origin only), whose diets were devoid of long chain fatty acids, and five omnivores (people who eat all types of food). The linseed oil supplement which contained linolenic acid led to a very small increase in the proportion of fatty acid in platelet plasma phosphoglycerides of the omnivores and even smaller increase in the vegans, whose diet was rich in linoleic acid.

When the omnivore subjects were given a supplement of EPA there was a dramatic increase in the long chain fatty acids in plasma and platelet phosphoglycerides and a corresponding reduction in the proportion of arachidonic acid and docosatetraenoic acid. This shows clearly that fish oil was far more potent in activity. Sanders also found that plasma triglyceride concentrations were reduced by the rich fish oil supplement but not by the linseed oil supplement.

In a subsequent study Sanders studied the influence of daily supplements of 5, 10 and 20 grams of EPA for three-week periods in five subjects. Even at the lowest level, the proportion of platelet phosphoglycerides was substantially increased. Triglyceride concentrations were reduced in all subjects taking 20 and 10 grams per day and in some subjects at 5 grams per day. However, platelet aggregation was not inhibited.

Sinclair subjected himself to an Eskimo diet for six weeks and showed a marked increase in bleeding time and reductions in platelet count and VLDL cholesterol.[24] His serum HDL rose and there were significant changes in plasma lipid fatty acid composition.

Saynor and Verel fed 20 milliliters of EPA for five weeks to volunteers and found a rise in HDL cholesterol and a fall in serum triglycerides but no significant change in total cholesterol, induced platelet aggregation, fibrinogen level, antithrombin III or thrombin time.[25] Kinsell et al. showed as long ago as 1961 that a fish oil compound of 5 or 6 double bonds could reduce serum lipid levels in diabetic patients even when consuming a normal allowance of saturated fat.[26] Cholesterol levels were also reduced by approximately 15 percent.

Kingsbury et al. fed volunteers on 50 grams of cod liver oil per day for up to 23 days.[19] They found a decrease in serum cholesterol concentration of approximately 27 percent. The serum cholesterol level rapidly rose when the cod liver oil supplement was discontinued. In a further experiment Kingsbury et al. fed 15 or 30 grams of cod liver oil for a four-week period to volunteers. At the end of this period, the mean plasma concentration of cholesterol had fallen by 8 percent and 18 percent respectively. Jakubowski had shown that platelet function can be modified by diet.[27]

Saynor and Verel extended their original observations to heart patients and found much the same results as in their earlier studies.[28]

Heart patients were involved in a much earlier trial of fish oil consumption. Nelson, a physician from Seattle, used a fish diet to treat heart patients as early as 1972.[29] The paper indicated a substantially longer survival for those patients who adhered to the regime, details of which were not given, compared with those who did not.

Saynor tested over 100 cardiac patients, many of whom originally had raised serum triglycerides, with an EPA supplement.[30] In virtually every case, the triglycerides decreased to within normal limits.

In a study conducted at the University of Oregon Health Sciences Center, Portland, using a ten-day diet of salmon which contains both

EPA and DHA, plasma cholesterol levels dropped by 17 percent in presumably healthy volunteers and by 20 percent or more in patients who had elevated cholesterol and mildly elevated triglyceride levels. The triglyceride levels fell by as much as 40 percent in healthy volunteers and by as much as 67 percent in those whose levels had been elevated originally.

## INCORPORATING EPA AND DHA INTO THE DIET

The evidence is that EPA and DHA are not efficiently produced in the human body, but must come from dietary sources to yield optimal health.

It is possible to do as one researcher did and adopt the eating habits of Eskimos.[24] However, it seems unlikely that many people will choose to do so. In fact, it seems clear that there is a limit to the number of times each week that one would want to eat fatty fish such as mackerel, salmon, sardines or anchovies. Of course, Americans did eat more fatty fish before the heart disease epidemic, but our tastes and calorie needs have changed.

Even the use of oils such as cod liver oil has a drawback: Many people strongly dislike the taste. Also, cod liver oil is high in vitamins A and D which limits the amount that can be safely taken. In addition, cod liver oil contains 20 and 22 carbon-chain, single-bond compounds which can cause an accumulation of fat and heart damage when consumed in large quantities.

EPA and DHA are available in capsule form in a commercial product called MaxEPA, that is both high in EPA and DHA and low in vitamins A and D. The trade name MaxEPA is available as several brands from various suppliers.

Sanders and Younger compared the effects of linseed oil supplement (an unsaturated oil which does not have omega-3 fatty acids) versus MaxEPA in both vegetarian and omnivorous subjects.[23] In both groups, the MaxEPA had a much stronger effect on lowering triglyceride levels and reducing platelet aggregation.

Dr. Sanders then conducted a study to examine the influence of daily

FISH OIL AND HEART ATTACKS

A study by Dr. Kenneth Radack of the University of Cincinnati School of Medicine suggests that even low doses of fish oil will reduce the risk of a heart attack. Dr. Radack believes that the oil either affects cholesterol levels or inhibits the formation of blood clots, which can precipitate a heart attack.

In the study, ten volunteers were given six capsules of fish oil daily, seven received three capsules, and eight were given olive oil. The researchers were especially concerned about blood levels of fibrinogen, a protein related to blood clotting.

After 20 weeks of this regimen, fibrinogen levels had dropped 21.6 percent in those receiving six fish oil capsules each day; it had dropped 5.8 percent in those given three capsules each day; there was no change in the olive oil group.

"Such reductions could have potential in lowering the risk for cardiovascular disease," Dr. Radack said. (*Annals of Internal Medicine,* November 1989.)

supplements of 5 grams, 10 grams, and 20 grams of MaxEPA for three-week periods in five subjects. Each experimental period was separated by at least six weeks. The results of this study showed that even at 5 grams per day, the level of EPA in the subjects' blood was substantially increased. Triglyceride levels were reduced in all subjects at 20 grams and 10 grams per day, and in some subjects at 5 grams per day.

Other formulations containing rich amounts of EPA and DHA will undoubtedly appear in the marketplace when clinical trials are conducted on those specific formulations.

## REFERENCES

1. Chief Medical Officer of Greenland. The State of Health in Greenland. Annual Reports for 1973–76. Denmark, Godthab. 1978.
2. Sinclair, H. M. Fats and Atheroma. *British Medical Journal.* 4/28/79, p. 69.

3. Kato. H.; Tillotson, J.; Nichamai, M. Z.; Rhoads, G. G.; Hamilton, H. B. Epidemiological Studies of Coronary Heart Disease and Stroke in Japanese Men Living in Japan, Hawaii and California: Serum Lipids and Diet. *American Journal of Epidemiology* 97. 6/73, pp. 372–385.
4. Lee, J. B. The Prostaglandins. *Textbook of Endocrinology,* 5th ed. edited by R. H. Williams. Philadelphia: W. B. Saunders Co., 1974.
5. Bennet, A. Prostaglandins. *Recent Advances in Clinical Pharmacology.* 1978, pp. 17–30.
6. Korsan-Bengsten, K., *et al.* Thrombosis Diathes. *Haemorrh.,* 1972.
7. Passwater, R. *Supernutrition for Healthy Hearts.* New York: Dial Press, 1977.
8. Gordon, T., *et al. Am. J. Med.* 62: 707–714, 1977.
9. Williams, P., *et al. Lancet* 1:72–75, 1979.
10. Hirai, A., *et al.* Eicosapentaenoic Acid and Platelet Function in Japanese. *Lancet* ii, 1980, p. 1132.
11. Sanders, T. A. B. Personal communication. 1/14/82.
12. Hirai, A. EPA and Platelet Function in Japanese. *Lancet* ii, 1980, p. 1132.
13. Sen, D. P. *et al.* Hypocholesteromic Effect Induced in Rats by Oil-Sardine Fish and Sardine Oils Having Different Degrees of Unsaturation. *JAOCS,* July 1977, 54, pp. 297–303.
14. Ruiter, A., *et al.* The Influence of Dietary Mackerel Oil on the Condition of Organs and on Blood Lipid Composition in Growing Pig. *Am. Jnl. Clin. Nutri.,* 12/78, 31, pp. 2159–2166.
15. Hornstra, G.; Haddeman, E.; Ten Hoor, F. Fish Oils, Prostaglandins and Arterial Thrombosis. *Lancet* 11/17/79.
16. Hornstra, G. and Hemker, H. C. Clot Promoting Effect of Platelet Vessel Wall Interactions: Influence of Dietary Fats and Relation to Arterial Thrombosis Formation in Rats. *Haemostasis,* 1979, 8, pp. 211–226.
17. Von Lossonczy, T. O.; Ruiter, A.; Hermus, R. J. J.; Van Gent, C. M.; Bronsgeest-Schoute, H. C. Effect of Fish Diet on Serum Lipids in Healthy Human Subjects. *Am. Jnl. Clin. Nutri.* 1978, 31, pp. 1340–1346.
18. Van Gent, C. M.; Luten, J. B.; Ruiter, A.; Bronsgeest-Schoute, H. C. Effect on Serum Lipid Levels of W-3 Fatty Acids of Ingesting Fish Oil Concentrate. *Lancet* 12/8/79, pp. 1249–1250.
19. Kingsbury, K. J.; Morgan, D. M.; Aylott, C.; Emmerson, R. Effects of Ethyl Arachidonate, Cod Liver Oil and Corn Oil on the Plasma Cholesterol Level. *Lancet,* 1961, i, p. 739.

20. Siess, W.; Roth, P.; Scherer, B. C.; Bohlig, B.; Weber, P. C. Platelet Membrane Fatty Acids, Platelet Aggregation and Thromboxane Formation during Mackerel Diet. *Lancet,* 3/15/80, pp. 441–444.
21. Harris, W. W. and Connor, W. E. The Effect of Salmon Oil upon Plasma Lipids, Lipoproteins and Triglyceride Clearance. *Trans. Assoc. Amer. Phys. xciii,* 1980, p. 148.
22. Dyerberg, J., Bang, H. O., Aagaard, O. Alpha Linolenic Acid and Eicosapentaenoic Acid. *Lancet,* 1/26/80, p. 199.
23. Sanders, T. A. B. and Younger, K. M. The Effect of Dietary Supplements of W-3 Polyunsaturated Fatty Acids on the Fatty Acid Composition of Platelets and Plasma Choline Phosphoglycerides. *British Journal of Nutrition,* 1981, 45, p. 613.
24. Sinclair, H. Advantages and Disadvantages of an Eskimo Diet. *Drugs Affecting Lipid Metabolism.* Arlington, Va: AFIPS Press, distributor for Elsevier North-Holland Inc. Biomedical Press, 1980.
25. Saynor, R. and Verel, D. Effect of a Marine Oil High in Eicosapentaenoic Acid on Blood Lipids and Coagulation. *I.R.C.S., Med. Sci.,* 1980, 8, pp. 378–379.
26. Kinsell, L. W.; Michaels, G. D.; Walker, G.; Visintine, R. E. The Effect of a Fish Oil Fraction of Plasma Lipids. *Diabetes,* 1961, 10 (4), pp. 316–319.
27. Jakubowski, J. A. and Ardlie, N. G. Modification of Human Platelet Function by a Diet Enriched in Saturated Fat or Polyunsaturated Fat. *Atherosclerosis,* 1978, 31, pp. 335–344.
28. Saynor, R. and Verel, D. Effect of a Fish Oil on Blood Coagulation. *Throm. Haem.,* 1981 (July), 46 (1), p. 65.
29. Nelson, A. M. Diet Therapy in Coronary Disease. *Geriatrics,* 1972 (December), pp. 103–116.
30. Saynor, R. Personal communication. 1981.

I am especially thankful for the several helpful discussions with Dr. Tom Sanders of Queen Elizabeth College, London. I am also grateful to Bob Fredericks and Sid Tracy of R.P. Scherer Corporation and to the Seven Seas Health Care Ltd. of Hull, England for responding to my many requests for information.

R. Passwater

# Omega-3 Fish Oils Shown To Reduce Hypertension

According to a study from the University of Nebraska's Department of Human Nutrition and Food Service Management in Lincoln, the omega-3 fatty acids found in certain fish can reduce high blood pressure. Results of the study were reported at the 198th national meeting of the American Chemical Society in Miami Beach, Florida, on September 11, 1989.

"Omega-3 fatty acids help to keep proper electrolyte balance in the body by causing excess sodium to be excreted in the urine, thereby reducing blood pressure," reported Constance Kies, Ph.D.

In the study, healthy volunteers were given 540 milligrams of omega-3 supplements daily for 28 days. Omega-3 is also available in such fish as tuna, salmon, halibut, lake trout, chub, herring, whitefish and smelt.

According to Dr. Kies, omega-3 works against high blood pressure by moderating biological activators in the body known as eicosanoids. These activators regulate all types of biological activities, including kidney function. When omega-3 becomes an eicosanoid inside the body, it interacts with other eicosanoids that are specific to kidney function and prevents them from allowing too much fluid retention and consequent abnormal sodium levels.

"Electrolyte balance has long been associated with hypertension and stroke, since electrolytes are supposed to keep the body's fluids in balance," Dr. Kies continued. "Since fluid follows sodium, it is attracted by sodium, and hypertensives often retain fluid rather than excreting it."

# FISH OILS

*Marine Lipids and Their Newly Discovered Health Roles*

RICHARD A. PASSWATER, PH.D.

A FISHY FUTURE

The omega-3 fatty acids EPA and DHA, found in coldwater fish, are producing a near-revolution in approaches to such conditions as heart disease, arthritis, diabetes, migraines and some forms of cancer. Definitive research is still being done, and the most exciting discoveries are yet to come, but the work surveyed here indicates strongly that good health and substantial fish and fish oil intake are closely linked.

## THE MANY BENEFITS OF FISH OILS

The amazing benefits of fish oils continue to be discovered by today's medical researchers. In 1982, when I wrote *EPA—Marine Lipids,*[1] the research indicated that fish oils could dramatically reduce heart disease, but the biochemistry concerning the interrelationships of fish oils, prostaglandins and health were so unknown to nutritionists and physicians that I had to devote much of the booklet to explaining the biochemistry involved.

Now fish oils are so widely recognized for their beneficial role in preventing and/or alleviating heart disease, high blood pressure, arthritis and migraine headaches that there is barely room to discuss these studies in this book. In addition, there is exciting research that shows that fish oils may be protective against cancer, immune deficiency diseases, kidney disease and others. So, in this essay, I will concentrate on practical health information.

When I wrote this material in 1987, there were several articles in the *New England Journal of Medicine* extolling the many benefits of fish oils, plus a front-page story in *USA Today* telling of still one more way in which fish oils protect the heart.

The knowledge involving the balancing of dietary oils to optimize prostaglandin production undoubtedly will lead to many more beneficial health discoveries in the near future. Therefore, I'll give a brief review of basics here, but those wanting more details about how fish oils make prostaglandins and how prostaglandins work to restore health can read Chapter 1, *EPA-Marine Lipids.*

## REVIEW OF BASIC FISH OIL BIOCHEMISTRY

Fish oils are of such great importance because they contain two special nutrients. These special nutrients form the compounds that protect the heart and arteries, reduce pain, inflammation and swelling and protect cell membranes. Strangely enough, these special nutrients belong to the *fat* family of nutrients. In spite of the fact that many people have too much fat overall in their diet, most people are lacking these special fats or they can't produce sufficient quantities of them from other dietary fats. Many researchers believe that most people are getting too much of the wrong kinds of fats, and need the fish oil fats to *balance* the family of fat nutrients.

Most people's diets have too many animal-source saturated fats and too many vegetable-source polyunsaturated fats. They should lower total fat intake to 20 to 30 percent of daily calorie intake, while appreciably increasing intake of the fats found in the oils of certain fish. In addition, a significant number of people will benefit from increasing the amount of still another fat called *gamma-linolenic acid* (GLA).*

The point is that fat is not fat is not fat! Just as there are different vitamins and different amino acids, with each having their own metabolic tasks, there are different fats which have different body functions. We have learned not to think only in terms of vitamin A and protein, but in terms of a balance of all vitamins and amino acids. Now we should learn to think in terms of a balance of all fat groups.

As an example of the effect of different fats on health and lifespan, consider the study by Dr. A. Bennett at Ball State University in Muncie, Indiana.[2] Mice were fed a high-fat diet rich in either the polyunsaturated fatty acid linoleic acid, the primary fat in vegetable oils, or the saturated fatty acid stearic acid, the primary fat in beef. The average lifespan of mice fed the linoleic acid-rich diet was less than 20 months, while the average lifespan of mice fed the saturated fat was more than 30 months. No, that's not a typo, the mice lived more than 50 percent longer on the saturated animal fat diet than on the polyunsaturates. Yet many people are being urged to eat more polyunsaturated, rather than saturated fats.

The significant point is that fats are different and different dietary fats may have varying effects on health and lifespan.

Oils and fats are both members of the same chemical family called lipids. Actually the word "fat" is an acceptable word for nonchemists to use in place of "lipid." It is also acceptable to call lipids that are solid at room temperature fats, and lipids that are liquid at room temperature, oils.

The number of atoms in each molecule and the degree of saturation of each molecule help to determine whether a lipid is solid or liquid at room temperature.

Fish oils and vegetable oils are both made up of largely *polyunsaturated fatty acids* (PUFA). Fatty acids are the basic units of fats. Typical body fats are formed by joining three fatty acids to a frame of

*Gamma-linolenic acid is an important fatty acid found in human milk, evening primrose oil, black currants, borage oil and a few other foods. The importance of GLA to nutrition and health is discussed in the chapter on Evening Primrose Oil.

*glycerol.* Basically, there are two major families of PUFA: the omega-6 (w-6 or n-6) family and the omega-3 (w-3 or n-3) family; and one major family of monounsaturated fatty acids, the omega-9 (w-9 or n-9). The difference between the families is in the position of the double bonds. In omega-3 fats, the first double bond is three carbon atoms from the terminal end (omega) of the molecule; in omega-6 fats, it's six carbon atoms, and so on. Chemists consider the methyl group to be the end of the fatty acid molecule and the carboxyl acid group to be the beginning of the molecule.

The major dietary source of the omega-6 family is linoleic acid (LA). In modern Western diets the major source of the omega-3 family is alpha-linolenic acid (ALA). In societies having low incidence of heart disease, the major dietary sources of the omega-3 family are often eicosapentaenoic acid (EPA) and docosahexaenoic acid (DHA). The major source of the omega-9 family is oleic acid.

The major dietary fatty acids can, to some extent, be converted in the body to other fatty acids that are needed for various functions, particularly the production of prostaglandins (PGs), hormone-like compounds having great biologic influence. PGs are regulators that are manufactured in the cells at the point of use, rather than being produced in a distant gland and having to be transported in the bloodstream to where they will be used.

PGs are not stored, and are quickly inactivated by enzymes. Each tissue makes PGs as needed, if the appropriate fatty acid precursors are present in the tissues in adequate quantities. Some organ systems depend on a balance of PGs which act in opposing ways.

Prostaglandins are so named because the first one was isolated in the prostate gland. They control or influence many body processes, including blood pressure, blood clotting, blood sugar, menstrual cramps, gastrointestinal secretion, fertility, reproduction, immunity, inflammation and pain. These functions are involved in heart disease, arthritis, asthma, migraine headaches, glaucoma, diabetes, cancer and other disorders. Some of the functions are desirable, some are not. Desirable functions are usually controlled by the PGs of the PG1 and PG3 family.

The PG1 family is produced from GLA, while the PG3 family is produced from EPA and DHA. The abundant PG2 family is produced from LA and arachidonic acid (AA), both of vegetable source. PG2s produce some desirable functions, as well as several undesirable functions. LA and AA also produce compounds related to PGs that are not desirable.

The conversion of LA to GLA and the conversion of ALA to EPA or DHA are hindered by the wrong diet, illness and aging. The wrong diet, too little of certain vitamins and minerals, and too much saturated fat block the conversion.

Therefore, many individuals do not have optimal stores of EPA, DHA and GLA and cannot produce optimal amounts of PG3 and PG1. Their prostaglandin production is unbalanced towards PG2, and they tend to have "sticky" blood, membrane problems, inflammation and other difficulties.

For your information, and not to make a big issue of the various types of PGs, it should be pointed out that there are several family members of PGs within each of the PG1, PG2 and PG3 families. They are designated by another letter, such as an "E" or an "F" following the "PG" and before the number. Scientists have identified more than twenty different PGs. Of these, the members designated as PGEs, PGFs and PGIs are the most important.

This may be more than you ever wanted to know about fatty acids and PGs. It is presented for your information, but you certainly don't have to understand all that chemical jargon to understand the test results and facts about how fish oil protects against all those diseases. It will help you to understand why fish oil works, but we used aspirin for a century before we understood how it worked. (Which, by the way, turns out to be via its influence on PGs.)

The key is a balance of the PGs and the dietary fats. While stressing the importance of EPA, DHA and GLA and emphasizing their disparity in the diet, keep in mind that LA still is an important dietary factor. The daily diet should contain about 3 grams of LA. As Dr. J. Kinsella points out in *Nutrition Today,* "no other nutrient affects so many physiological interactions as does LA via its conversion to

AA and thence to [PG2 and related compounds]."[3] However, Americans average about 25 grams of LA, which far exceeds the requirement and actually becomes a problem because some of the products formed from LA interfere with the conversion to desirable PGs.

## HEART DISEASE

In *EPA—Marine Lipids,* covering research through mid-1982, I described the epidemiological research that gave scientists the clue that there might be some factor in fish oil that protected the Eskimos from heart disease. Eskimos eat a very high-fat diet and according to conventional wisdom would be expected to have a very high incidence of heart disease instead of their actual very low rate. When Europeans normally eating a Westernized diet were switched to an Eskimo-like diet high in cold-water fish, the European volunteers had changes in their blood that are associated with protection against heart attacks.

Low death rates from heart disease are also found in Japan, where fish intake is very high. Within Japan, the lowest heart disease death rate is found on the island of Okinawa, where fish consumption is about twice as high as on the mainland. In a study in the Chiba Prefecture, residents of fishing villages had lower heart disease death rates than those living in farming villages. Fish consumption in the fishing village averaged about 9 ounces compared to about 3.2 ounces in the farming villages.

Follow-up experiments with fish oil, first in laboratory animals and then in clinical trials, found the same changes in blood chemistry—blood that was more free-flowing or less sticky that tended not to clot as easily. Blood that clots too easily is prone to collect in narrowed coronary arteries and shut off the blood flow to the heart. This is called a heart attack or coronary thrombosis, and results in heart tissue destruction, which is called myocardial infarction.

Other beneficial changes to the blood produced by fish oil noted by the researchers were lowered cholesterol and triglyceride levels.

Laboratory animal experiments continued to broaden our knowledge and add more mechanisms showing how fish oils reduce heart attacks. In November 1982, researchers at the University of Michigan Medical School demonstrated that fish oil decreases the reactivity of blood vessels to stress hormones.[4]

A small-scale clinical study in Japan indicated that EPA reduced TXB2 (a thromboxane that can cause clotting), platelet aggregation (a measure of blood's tendency to clot) and blood viscosity. The researchers concluded that EPA produces no side effects and may be useful in the treatment and prevention of thrombotic diseases—disease involving blood clotting as is the case in most heart attacks.[5]

## CHOLESTEROL AND TRIGLYCERIDES

The Harris-Connor group examined the effect of fish oil on high-carbohydrate diets. These diets increase the blood levels of very-low-density lipoproteins (VLDL) and triglycerides. VLDL are carriers that transport mostly triglycerides and some cholesterol in the blood. They are smaller than the more familiar low-density lipoproteins (LDL) and high-density lipoproteins (HDL). It is well recognized that having more HDL than LDL protects against heart disease. The role of VLDL is not as well understood, but some researchers feel that high levels of VLDL are also a risk factor in heart disease.

The studies compared the effects of fish oils and plant oils on the blood levels of VLDL and triglycerides in healthy persons eating a high-carbohydrate diet. The healthy volunteers were placed on a diet that was 45 percent carbohydrate and 45 percent fat for a period of time to establish baseline measurements. Next they were placed on a 75 percent carbohydrate diet, 15 percent of which consisted of peanut oil and cocoa butter. (Either that tastes better than I think, or we have here an example of self-sacrifice in the cause of science!) After a period of time, the plant fats were replaced with fish oils, while the remainder of the diet was unchanged.

When the volunteers consumed the high-carbohydrate diet without the fish oils, their blood levels of triglycerides rose an average of 85 percent while their VLDL more than doubled. But when they were switched to the high-carbohydrate diet with fish oils, their blood level of triglycerides dropped from the elevated level to a level that was even lower than the baseline level associated with the moderate-carbohydrate diet. Their average VLDL level dropped 78 percent and the cholesterol level dropped 65 percent to below baseline level. These effects were seen within three days of adding fish oil to the diet.[6,7]

In 1985, members of this research group reported that fish oils produced dramatic drops in blood triglyceride levels in patients having highly elevated levels of these fats. Fish oils were far more effective than corn oil or safflower oil.[8]

A study from Karlovy University in Prague, Czechoslovakia also showed that fish oils reduced high triglycerides. Men with elevated blood levels of triglycerides who were given about 18 ounces of fish daily for three months had reductions in triglyceride levels and improvements in HDL levels.[9]

In 1986, Dr. Paul Nestel of the Baker Medical Research Institute in Melbourne, Australia showed that adding fish oil to a high-cholesterol diet prevented increased blood cholesterol levels and possibly reduced the risk of heart disease. He fed volunteers three different diets over a seven-week period: a normal diet, a fish-oil diet, and a fish oil—egg yolk diet.

The normal diet had a PUFA-to-saturated fat ratio of 0.47 and a daily cholesterol level of 710 milligrams. The fish oil diet (40 grams of MaxEPA* per day) had a PUFA-to-saturated fat ratio of 1.62 and a daily cholesterol level of 190 milligrams. The fish oil-egg yolk diet had a PUFA-to-saturated fat ratio of 1.62 and a daily cholesterol level of 940 milligrams.

When the volunteers were switched from the normal diet to the fish oil diet, their blood cholesterol, VLDL, LDL, HDL and triglyceride levels declined. When they were then switched to the fish oil–egg

*MaxEPA is a trademark of Seven Seas Health Care Ltd., Hull, England; similar formulations include Promega, a trademark of the Parke-Davis Division of Warner-Lambert; and Proto-Chol a trademark of E. R. Squibb & Sons, Inc., Princeton, New Jersey.

yolk (high cholesterol) diet, the expected elevation in those blood components did not occur, however, cholesterol levels did rise slightly. It was concluded that fish oils are effective in lowering lipoprotein cholesterol levels even when the dietary intake of cholesterol is high.[10]

Following up on the laboratory findings reported in 1983, two studies confirmed that fish oils increase the time required for a blood clot to form by reducing the stickiness of the blood platelets that start the clotting mechanism in man as well as in laboratory animals.[11, 12]

## CORONARY MORTALITY

The studies of blood cholesterol and triglycerides are interesting, but do they really mean anything in terms of actual reduction in heart disease or is it just so much theory? To answer that question absolutely, long-term clinical trials are required. However, long-term retrospective studies and short-term prospective clinical trials are available and show significant evidence.

A series of articles and an editorial in the highly respected *New England Journal of Medicine* (NEJM) opened many eyes. Fish oils came of age on May 9, 1985 when these articles were published and were read by doctors who had not even heard of this research until then. One of the articles has already been discussed, but it applied only to the levels of blood components believed to be involved in the heart disease process. The real attention-grabber was an article from the Netherlands.

A research team at the University of Leiden's Institute of Social Medicine in the Netherlands, led by Dr. Daan Kromhout, produced the first long-term study of the effects of fish oils on heart disease deaths.

> We were aware of the low death rate from coronary heart disease among the Greenland Eskimos. We therefore decided

> to investigate the relation between fish consumption and coronary heart disease in a group of men in the town of Zutphen, the Netherlands. Information about the fish consumption of 852 middle-aged men without clinical signs or any other indication of coronary heart disease was collected in 1960 by a careful dietary history obtained from the participants and their wives.
>
> During twenty years of follow-up, 78 men died from coronary heart disease. An inverse dose-response relation was observed between the consumption in 1960 and the death from coronary heart disease during twenty years of follow-up. This relation persisted after factoring for other variables. Mortality from coronary heart disease was 58 percent lower among those who consumed at least 30 grams (slightly more than an ounce) of fish per day than among those who did not eat fish.
>
> We conclude that the consumption of as little as one or two fish dishes per week may be of preventive value in relation to coronary heart disease.[13]

The relationship existed throughout the time period. Twenty-seven men died from coronary heart disease between 1960 and 1970, 51 between 1971 and 1980. The more fish the men ate, the fewer deaths due to heart disease, and the lower the total death rate, as other diseases were not affected.

For those who worry too much about dietary cholesterol, it should be noted that the men eating the most fish also ate the most cholesterol and animal protein, yet had lower heart disease deaths. Please keep in mind the studies showing that fish and fish oils both tend to lower blood cholesterol levels, regardless of the dietary cholesterol content.

On September 26, 1985, *NEJM* published some of the letters it had received commenting on the three articles and the editorial in the May 9 issue. Among the responses was data from the group that conducted the Western Electric study on heart disease that began in 1957. When Drs. Jeremiah Stamler, Richard Shekelle, Oglesby Paul and their colleagues examined their data in terms of fish consumption versus heart disease death rate, they confirmed the Kromhout group's observations. The Western Electric data showed that the 25-year risk of death from coronary heart disease for those men consuming more than 35 grams of fish per day was only 65 percent of that for those who did not eat fish.[14]

Researchers led by Dr. Robert Wissler of the University of Chicago studied the effects of fish oil on the walls of arteries. They found that fish oil reduced plaque formation in rhesus monkeys, which have arteries and a biochemistry very similar to humans.

The researchers fed sixteen rhesus monkeys a diet high in fish oil, and fed a group of eight rhesus monkeys a diet similar except that it was high in saturated fat. The monkeys fed the fish oil diet not only developed fewer deposits in their arteries, but the deposits contained fewer inflammatory cells and were less likely to cause medical complications, according to Dr. Wissler. The monkeys fed the fish oil diet had lower blood levels of LDL cholesterol as well.[15]

And just when we think that we have learned all the ways in which fish oils protect us against death by heart attack, another one turns up! Dr. Carl Hock at the University of Medicine and Dentistry of New Jersey told researchers attending the 1986 annual meeting of the American Heart Association of experiments in which he fed a group of laboratory rats a diet with the predominant fat being fish oils and another group a diet with corn oil predominating.[16] After four weeks, he blocked the flow of blood to the rats' hearts. The rats that were fed fish oils had less tissue damage and less loss of an important enzyme usually destroyed during a heart attack.

He also found that EPA had become part of the heart's cell structure.

We have seen that fish oils reduce the heart disease death rate in people over periods of from 10 to 25 years, that fish oils reduce the development of coronary artery disease and protect the heart against damage from heart attack. It was also reassuring to note that fish oils reduced the blood levels of factors that are associated with the risk of heart disease. But there is still more to the story.

## BLOOD PRESSURE

High blood pressure is called a "silent killer" because it produces no pain or symptoms, yet it is a major risk factor for stroke and other diseases of the arteries. The good news is that fish oils, at least some of them, help normalize blood pressure.

Physicians at the Central Institute for Cardiovascular Research in the German Democratic Republic reported in July 1985 that a mackerel diet containing 2.2 grams of EPA daily produced a significantly lower systolic (upper number) blood pressure in eight of eight patients having an inherited disorder that produces abnormally high blood triglyceride and cholesterol levels and premature heart disease. The disease is called familial hyperlipoproteinemia. The mackerel diet also reduced blood cholesterol and triglycerides for a period of three months, after which they tended to drift back towards their previous values, as is the usual case with these patients and dietary modification.[17]

Later this research group studied fourteen patients having moderate high blood pressure (*essential hypertension*). The mackerel diet decreased systolic blood pressure by almost 10 percent. Whenever the subjects were returned to their normal diets, their blood pressure increased again. When they were again given the mackerel diet, their blood pressure dropped towards normal.

Other blood parameters associated with high blood pressure were also improved. Blood sodium (salt) levels decreased and renin (a hormone produced in the kidney that greatly affects blood pressure) activity increased by 64 percent. The researchers concluded that these data suggest a beneficial effect of a mackerel diet on patients with mild essential hypertension.[18]

In 1986, researchers at the London Chest Hospital studied 16 patients having mild hypertension. They were given MaxEPA fish oil capsules for 12 weeks in a placebo controlled, cross-over study. Their blood pressure averaged 160/94 at the start of the study. After being on a placebo for six weeks, their blood pressures remained at an average of 161/94.5 as would be expected. However, after being switched to MaxEPA fish oil capsules for six weeks, their blood pressures dropped to an average of 151/92.5. The drop in systolic pressure was statistically significant.

Most patients reported that they preferred the fish oil supplements to their previous treatment. The researchers concluded that fish oil supplementation may provide a safe, more acceptable treatment for patients with mild essential systolic hypertension who are reluctant to embark on drug therapies.[19]

## OTHER SEVERE HEALTH CONDITIONS

Heart disease is what aroused scientific interest in fish oils, but now that we are beginning to understand the biochemistry involved we are seeing that EPA can benefit a host of health problems.

### ARTHRITIS AND LUPUS

Animal studies at Harvard indicated that EPA helps protect the body against attack by its own immune system in *autoimmune* diseases such as rheumatoid arthritis and lupus erythematosus.[20, 21]

The researchers were studying the effects of EPA on the inflammatory process and kidney disease. They reasoned that, if EPA reduces the body's production of inflammatory compounds, it should aid arthritis and lupus sufferers. A key factor in the inflammation process is *leukotriene* B4 (LTB4). LTB4 can make a major contribution to joint discomfort and pain. Tissues can make LTB4 out of omega-6 fatty acids, but when omega-3 fatty acid EPA is present, leukotriene B5 (LTB5) is made instead. LTB5 is relatively benign in comparison to LTB4.

A 1985 article in *Clinical Research* reported that fish oil supplements significantly improved the health of rheumatoid arthritis patients. Dr. Joel M. Kremer, an associate professor of medicine at

Albany Medical College, and his colleagues reported a 40-patient, placebo-controlled, double-blind, cross-over study.[22] They gave 15 MaxEPA capsules daily to 20 patients for 14 weeks. The patients continued their normal diets with the only difference being the MaxEPA supplement. At the same time another group of 20 arthritis patients took the same number of placebo capsules.

After the 14-week period, all 40 patients began a four-week washout period in which they took no MaxEPA or placebo. The groups were then "cross-overed," i.e., each group then took the capsules formerly taken by the other group, for 14 weeks. Another four-week washout period followed. Thirty-three patients completed the clinical trial. Dr. Kremer reports, "Those taking fish oil had only about half the number of tender joints as they had prior to the study, and about half as many as the patients taking the placebo. The benefit vanished during the washout period." The researchers also noted that MaxEPA slowed the onset of fatigue.

Dr. Kremer also gave an updated report on the study at the 1986 annual meeting of the American Rheumatism Association (ARA), in which he reported that MaxEPA produced a 60-percent reduction in LTB4 in humans as well as laboratory animals, and increased the production of LTB5 in humans. Dr. Kremer reported, "We saw a significant correlation between the drop in leukotriene B4 and the decrease in the number of tender joints. Those receiving the EPA supplement weren't in as much pain, their joints were less tender and they made it through the day longer before fatigue set in."

Dr. Dwight R. Robinson, a rheumatologist at Massachusetts General Hospital, reported that MaxEPA has the most striking protective effect seen thus far in any animal tests of inflammatory diseases. He found that MaxEPA was effective in laboratory mice having systemic lupus. The National Institutes of Health is conducting further research on lupus patients.

## MIGRAINES

There is even good news about fish oil for migraineurs—migraine sufferers.

Fish oil dramatically reduces the frequency and severity of migraine headaches, according to studies at the University of Cincinnati Medical Center. Dr. Charles J. Glueck and his associates conducted a 19-week, double-blind; placebo-crossover controlled, clinical trial involving eight women and seven men; severe classic migraineurs who had not responded to any of the gamut of antimigraine therapy that they received. They were given either 15 grams of MaxEPA or placebo for six weeks, followed by a three-week placebo washout period, and then "crossed over" for six weeks to the opposite formulation.[22]

In males, MaxEPA significantly reduced migraines. In females, there was no significant difference between MaxEPA and the placebo. There was a significant reduction in headaches for the entire group. Five of the seven men had a greater than 33-percent reduction in headache score, while only two of eight women had a reduction in excess of 33 percent.

The researchers concluded that "the migraine ameliorating action of MaxEPA may be mediated through changes in prostaglandin synthesis and/or by reductions in platelet serotonin release, with an aggregate diminution in cerebral vasospasm." The researchers noted that nutritional supplementation with fish oil is a promising way to relieve migraine pain. It can benefit migraineurs who have not responded to drug therapy, who don't like to take medication, or who have severe reactions to migraine medications.

## CANCER

Research also suggests that diets high in fish oils may help prevent and arrest growth of breast, colon, prostate and pancreatic cancers. Dr. Rashida Karmali of Rutgers University and Memorial Sloan-Kettering Hospital has found that fish oil counteracts the action of vegetable oils that promote harmful cell changes.

In Dr. Karmali's studies, which were reported to the 1986 annual meeting of the American Dietetic Association in Las Vegas, rats given corn oil were compared to those given corn oil plus fish oil. Those given the fish oil had significantly fewer and smaller breast tumors. Dr. Karmali's colon and prostate experiments indicate that fish oil is also protective against those cancers.

In an earlier study, Dr. Karmali's group had shown that EPA inhibited the growth of transplanted tumors (mammary, adenocarcinoma). MaxEPA was given orally to laboratory rats for one week before and three weeks after they received the transplants of cancer tissue. The laboratory animals were maintained on standard laboratory diets, with the exception that different groups were given different amounts of EPA. After three weeks, tumor growth was significantly less in the three MaxEPA groups than in the unsupplemented controls.

Levels of AA were higher in tumors from laboratory animals given MaxEPA, and levels of prostaglandin and thromboxane products of AA metabolism were reduced. Tumor microsomes from animals given MaxEPA had decreased ability to synthesize AA metabolites. The researchers concluded that inhibition of AA metabolism may be a mammary cancer-reducing mechanism.[23]

In a study at Cornell University, rats injected with a chemical known to cause pancreatic cancer had fewer and smaller tumors with fish oil than with corn oil.[24] Dr. T. P. O'Connor and his colleagues concluded: "This study provides evidence that fish oils, rich in omega-3 fatty acids, may have potential as inhibitory agents in cancer development."

In a similar experiment, fish oil again proved to be an effective protector against cancer. Drs. J. Jurkowski and W. Cave of St. Mary's Hospital in Rochester used menhaden fish oil as the EPA source and N-methyl-N-nitrosourea as the cancer-causing chemical. The laboratory rats given fish oil survived an average of 38 percent longer, had 75 percent fewer tumors, and total tumor mass was 80 percent less than those not getting the fish oil.

All animals on their normal diets developed cancer, whereas 37.5

percent of rats given fish oil remained free of cancer. When corn oil was added to the normal diets, there was no significant change, and all of the rats developed cancer. Analysis of relevant tissues confirmed that EPA levels were inversely related to tumor development.[25]

It is thus apparent that cancer protection is a function of prostaglandin balance, not polyunsaturation. In fact, polyunsaturation from the omega-6 family—the LA from corn oil and other vegetable oils—is suspected of being a contributor to cancer development when the omega-6 PUFAs become excessive. Antioxidants such as vitamins A, C and E, plus the trace mineral selenium, are needed to counteract the excess of vegetable oils in today's diets. The cancer rate would drop dramatically if, on the average, vegetable oil consumption (but not whole vegetables) would drop, antioxidant nutrient consumption would increase, and EPA intake would increase.

If you are still unconvinced that the difference in the PUFA family and balance of PGs are not critical factors in cancer development, consider the following experiment.

Drs. H. Gabor and S. Abraham fed laboratory mice diets containing 10 percent fat from corn oil, menhaden fish oil, or hydrogenated cottonseed oil (hydrogen has been added to the molecule to change *unsaturated* bonds to saturated bonds). Cancer tissue—mammary adenocarcinomas—were transplanted into the mice, and tumors were weighed 21 days later. Tumors in mice fed fish oil or hydrogenated cottonseed oil were 60 percent smaller than those in mice fed corn oil.

The smaller tumor weights were due to increased rate of tumor cell loss, which was 2.5 times greater in mice fed fish oil than in those fed corn oil. The researchers concluded that omega-3 fatty acids contained in fish oils inhibit the stimulation of tumor growth induced by LA by altering prostaglandin synthesis.[26]

### DIABETES

It is not surprising that fish oils are beneficial to diabetics because they reduce heart and artery diseases that are associated with diabetes. However, recent research has also shown that fish oil helps non-insulin dependent diabetics (type 2) utilize their own insulin. Type 2 diabetics frequently develop the disease as a result of obesity and their insulin loses some of its effect in controlling blood sugar. Dutch researchers have found that 30 grams of MaxEPA daily improves type 2 diabetics' blood sugar control.[27]

Dr. Margaret J. Albrink, professor of medicine at West Virginia University in Morgantown, examined whether the beneficial cardiovascular effects of fish oils applied to diabetics as well.[28] She found that very large amounts of fish oil (45 milliliters, which contain nearly 18 grams of the omega-3 fatty acids) produced dramatic reductions of blood triglycerides and cholesterol, and returned *platelet* aggregation to normal without changing the bleeding time.

The above studies are just a sample of the exciting research that indicates there are considerable health benefits to normalizing prostaglandin levels by increasing the amount of fish in our diets. There is also research activity in psoriasis, multiple sclerosis, vision disorders, kidney disease and brain function.

## CONCLUSION

Research articles are being published at an ever-increasing rate. The National Institutes of Health are even advertising for researchers to apply for funds to further test and expand our knowledge about EPA. Most scientific publications have now carried news articles and editorials about fish oils, in addition to the research articles they publish. Even the Food and Drug Administration has published a favorable article in its *FDA Consumer* magazine.[29] The health advantages of adding fish oils to the diet are obvious. The question now becomes how to best do this.

## INCREASING DIETARY FISH OIL

It is unlikely that Americans will adopt the Eskimo diet, but there is no need to do so. Having one or two fish servings per week will please many people and convince the skeptics about the taste and meal variety that fish offer. Others may not prefer to do this and will opt to eat more fish on a regular basis and also include fish oil capsules as dietary supplements.

Please keep in mind that deep-frying fish will destroy the EPA and DHA. Broiling is a better method, and many feel that it improves the taste as well.

Table 1 lists the EPA and DHA content of selected foods, while Table 2 gives the total omega-3 fatty acid content of various fish and shellfish. Table 3 shows the amounts of fish, shellfish and supplements which supply one gram of EPA and DHA.

Fish oil supplements are available in a variety of forms, such as salmon oil, MaxEPA, Promega and Proto-Chol.* MaxEPA is a trade name of a blend of fish oils that has been commercially available for some time and has been used extensively in scientific research. MaxEPA is distributed by many supplement companies under their own label. It contains 18 percent EPA and 12 percent DHA. MaxEPA contains no fish liver oil so large amounts can be taken without appreciably increasing body vitamin A and D levels. Promega contains 35 percent EPA and 15 percent DHA.

The omega-3 fatty acids include those with shorter chains that may not be converted in the body to EPA or DHA. Some legumes, vegetables, plant oils, nuts and seeds also may contain omega-3 fatty acids, but no study reported to date has shown that consumption of the shorter-chain omega-3 fatty acids such as linolenic acid can produce the physiologic effect of marine omega-3 fatty acids.

Some physicians have suggested that vegetable sources of omega-3 fatty acids could be added to the diet, but studies have shown that

*MaxEPA is a trademark of Seven Seas Health Care Ltd., Hull, England; Promega is a trademark of the Parke-Davis Division of Warner-Lambert; Proto-Chol is a trademark of E. R. Squibb & Sons, Inc., Princeton, New Jersey.

TABLE 1. EPA AND DHA CONTENT OF SELECTED FOODS

| *Food (3.5 oz.)* | *Fat (grams)* | *EPA/DHA (grams)* | *Cholesterol (milligrams)* | *Calories* |
|---|---|---|---|---|
| Cod | 0.7 | 0.2 | 37 | 82 (steamed)<br>204 (fried) |
| Flounder | 1.0 | 0.2 | 46 | 53 (steamed)<br>214 (fried) |
| Salmon | 6.6 | 1.0–1.4 | 74 | 199 (steamed) |
| Trout | 3.4 | 0.5 | 57 | 131 (steamed) |
| Crab | 1.3 | 0.4 | 78 | 127 (boiled) |
| Lobster | 0.9 | 0.2 | 95 | 119 (boiled) |
| Shrimp | 1.3 | 0.2 | 128 | 114 (boiled) |

*Compiled from* USDA Handbook No. 8.

only EPA and DHA have produced the results discussed in this book. ALA is an omega-3, but it cannot be converted in adequate quantities, to EPA, which is needed to form the PG3 family of prostaglandins. Purslane, walnut oil, walnuts, wheat germ oil, canola oil (rapeseed oil that has had the theruic acid removed), soybean lecithin, soybeans and tofu, common beans, butternuts and seaweed are all fine foods, but they are not important sources of EPA and DHA.

A few physicians thought that it was better to have a vegetable source of EPA because fish sources have cholesterol in them. Now is this cholesterol phobia at its best—or its worst? EPA lowers cholesterol. The same MaxEPA supplements that worry a few anti-cholesterol people are the factors that lowered blood cholesterol levels. It is the blood cholesterol level—and even more important, the ratio of HDL to LDL cholesterol—that is important as a risk factor in heart disease.

A MaxEPA capsule that contains 180 milligrams of EPA and 120 mg of DHA contains only 5 mg of cholesterol, 10 calories, and 50 IU of vitamin A. To get the same amount of EPA from salmon, one would have to eat 30 grams, which would also contain 25 mg of

TABLE 2. TOTAL OMEGA-3 FATTY ACID CONTENT

| *Food (3.5 oz.)* | *Omega-3 (gram)* | *Total fat (gram)* |
|---|---|---|
| Salmon, Atlantic | 1.4 | - |
| Salmon, Pink | 1.0–1.9 | 5.2 |
| Salmon, Chinook, canned | 3.0 | 16.0 |
| Salmon, sockeye | 1.3 | 8.6 |
| Trout | 1.1–2.0 | 4.5 |
| Sardines | 2.9 | - |
| Mackerel | 2.2–2.6 | 9.8–13.9 |
| Herring | 1.1–1.7 | 6.2–9.0 |
| Tuna, canned | 1.5–1.7 | 6.6–6.8 |
| Anchovy | 1.4 | - |
| Bluefish | 1.2 | 6.5 |
| Halibut | 0.5–0.9 | 2.0 |
| Sablefish | 1.4 | 13.1 |
| Bass | 0.6 | 2.2 |
| Catfish | 0.6 | 3.6 |
| Perch | 0.5 | 2.5 |
| Haddock | 0.2 | 0.7 |
| Flounder | 0.3 | 1.2 |
| Hake | 0.6 | 2.6 |
| Mullet | 1.1 | 4.4 |
| Pompano | 0.6 | 9.5 |
| Shark | 0.5 | 1.9 |
| Swordfish | 0.2 | 2.1 |
| Oyster | 0.4–0.8 | 2.3–2.5 |
| Crab, Alaska king | 0.6 | 1.6 |
| Crab, blue, canned | 0.4–0.5 | 1.3–1.6 |
| Shrimp | 0.3–0.4 | 1.1–1.2 |

*Compiled from* The New England Journal of Medicine *316:625, March 5, 1987.*

cholesterol (five times that in MaxEPA) and 70 calories (seven times that of MaxEPA).

The safety and benefits have been studied here. It seems to be very wise for the average person to add fish to their diet. However, some people may be allergic to fish or have a medical problem that precludes them from doing this. By all means check with your doctor.

TABLE 3. QUANTITIES NEEDED TO SUPPLY 1 GRAM OF EPA AND DHA

| *Food* | *Grams* | *EPA and DHA (grams)* | *Cholesterol (milligrams)* | *Calories* |
|---|---|---|---|---|
| Cod | 500 | 1 | 185 | 410 |
| | | | | 1020 |
| Flounder | 500 | 1 | 230 | 265 |
| | | | | 1070 |
| Salmon | 100 | 1 | 74 | 199 |
| Trout | 200 | 1 | 114 | 262 |
| Crab | 250 | 1 | 195 | 317 |
| Lobster | 500 | 1 | 475 | 595 |
| Shrimp | 500 | 1 | 640 | 570 |
| MaxEPA | 3 | 1 | 14 | 27 |
| Cod liver oil | 5 | 1 | 25 | 45 |

*Compiled from the* Journal of the American Dietetic Association *86:788, 1986.*

## REFERENCES


1. Passwater, R. A. *EPA—Marine Lipids.* New Canaan, Connecticut: Keats Publishing, Inc., 1982.
2. Bennett, A. *et al. Gerontology* 26:74A, 1986.
3. Kinsella, J. E. *Nutr. Today* 7–14, Nov.-Dec., 1986.
4. Lockette, W. E. *et al. Prostaglandins* 24:631–8, Nov. 1982.
5. Terano, T. *et al. Atherosclerosis* 46:321–31, March 1983.
6. Harris, W. S. *et al. Metabolism* 32:179–84, 1983.
7. Harris, W. S. *et al. Metabolism* 33:1016–19, 1984.
8. Phillipson. B. E. *et al. New England J. Med.* 312:1210–16, May 9, 1985.
9. Chochola, M. *et al. Sb Lekar* 87:23–8, 1985.
10. Nestel, P. J. *Am. J. Clin. Nutr.* 43:752–757, 1986.
11. von Schacky, C. *et al. J. Clin. Invest.* 76:1626–31, 1985.
12. Knapp, H. R., *et al. NEJM* 314:937–42, 1986.
13. Kromhout, D., *et al. NEJM.* 312:1205–9, 1985.
14. Shekelle, R. B. *et al. NEJM* 313(13) 820, Sept. 26, 1985.
15. Anon. Nutrition Digest. *Prevention,* p. 100, April 1987.
16. Foley, E. *USA Today,* p. 1, March 4, 1987.

17. Singer, P. *et al. Atherosclerosis* 56:111–18, July 1985.
18. Ibid. 56:223–35, Aug. 1985.
19. Norris, P. G. *et al. British Med. J.* 293:104–5, July 12, 1986.
20. Lee, T. H. *et al. NEJM* 312(19) 1217–24, May 9, 1985.
21. Kremer, J. *et al. Clin. Res.* 33: A778, 1985.
22. Glueck, C. J. *et al. Am. J. Clin. Nutr.* In press, 1986.
23. Karmali, R. A. *et al. J. Nat. Cancer Inst.* 73:457–61, Aug. 1984.
24. O'Connor, T. P. *et al. J. Nat. Cancer Inst.* 75(5) 959–62, Nov. 1985.
25. Jurkowski, J. J. and Cave, W.T. *J. Natl. Cancer Inst.* 74:1145–50, May 1985.
26. Gabor, H. and Abraham, S. *J. Nat. Cancer Inst.* 76:1223–29, June 1986.
27. *Netherlands J. Med.* 29(2), 1986.
28. Albrink, M. J. *et al.* Annual Meeting of the American Diabetes Association, Anaheim, CA, 1986.
29. Zamula, E. *FDA Consumer* 20(8) 6–8, Oct. 1986.

# Fishing For Better Health?

## *You May Avoid Heart Disease And Cancer; Relieve Arthritis, Psoriasis With Fish Oils*

Interest in fish oils began to heat up in 1970, when Danish researchers found that Greenland Eskimos had a very low rate of heart disease, in spite of their traditional high-fat, high-cholesterol diet. In studying records from 1963 to 1967, the researchers determined that only two cases of atherosclerotic heart disease had occurred among the 1,300 inhabitants of an Eskimo settlement. One patient was 78 years old and the other one was suffering from rheumatic heart disease. In fact, heart disease mortality among Greenland Eskimos was only 3.5 percent of all deaths (as compared to 45.3 percent in the United States).

Since then, researchers from around the world have reported that fish oils—rich in omega-3 fatty acids—protect against cardiovascular disease and high blood pressure, lower the risk of colon cancer, relieve arthritis and other inflammatory disorders, prevent and treat some forms of cancer and kidney disease and ameloriate psoriasis and other skin problems. The only negative reports seem to be that fish oils may not be the proper treatment for some diabetics, and there are scattered reports that large amounts of fish oil may deplete vitamin E stores.

Researchers at the Jewish Hospital in Cincinnati, Ohio, reported in the *American Journal of Clinical Nutrition* (53:562–572, 1991) that both fish oil and corn oil lowered the blood pressure of elderly patients; however, the fish oils had the added advantage of lowering triglycerides, which in some patients may be more dangerous than cholesterol.

Which is best: fish or fish oil? The benefits of both were documented by researchers at the Division of Human Nutrition in South Australia, but the consumption of fish provides more benefits in the prevention and treatment of cardiovascular disease, they said. Both fish and fish oil capsules reduced triglycerides in the blood by 20 and 28 percent respectively, while raising high-density lipoprotein cholesterol by 10 and 9 percent respectively. However, fish oil did not reduce total cholesterol, low-density lipoprotein cholesterol, blood pressure or apolipoprotein B, according to their report in the *American Journal of Clinical Nutrition* (53:1210–1216, 1991).

## CONSIDER RATIO

In the January 1992 issue of *The Nutrition Report,* Elizabeth Somer, M.A., R.D. quoted Dr. A. Simopoulos at the Center for Genetics, Nutrition and Health in Washington, D.C. as recommending that the ratio of fats, such as the omega-3 and the omega-6 fatty acids, must be considered when making dietary recommendations. The reason, she said, that these two classes of polyunsaturated fatty acids should be distinguished is because they are metabolically and functionally distinct, as well as having opposing physiological functions.

"Perhaps the ill-fitting pieces in the fish oils story actually are components of a much broader puzzle," Somer said. "The modern human physique most closely resembles the prehistoric cave-dweller's body, which consumed a diet much lower in saturated fat and with small but roughly equal amounts of omega-3 and omega-6 fatty acids. This balance between fatty acids with a low total fat intake is probably more attuned to optimal serum lipids than in putting all the blame or fame on fish oils."

Preliminary research indicates that fish oils may be useful in the treatment of psoriasis, stated Robert H. Garrison, Jr., M.A., R.Ph. and Elizabeth Somer in *The Nutrition Desk Reference* (Keats Publishing, New Canaan, Conn. 1990). Symptoms improved when patients took a daily supplement of fish oil, which seems to reduce the blood levels of leukotrienes. These chemicals affect the inflammatory process and progression of psoriasis, they said.

Eicosapentaenoic acid (EPA), the fatty acid in fish oils, might be an effective therapy for the treatment of rheumatoid arthritis, the authors continued. Some patients have reported improvements in morning stiffness after taking fish oil.

"Omega-3 fatty acids compete with the omega-6 fatty acids, such as linoleic acid, and partially inhibit the production of some potent inflammatory mediators in the leukotriene and prostaglandin families," the authors said. "These biologically active substances produce very potent inflammatory agents that contribute to the painful reaction in the joints of patients with rheumatoid arthritis . . . In addition, patients with rheumatoid arthritis might require lower doses of antiinflammatory medications if dietary intake of omega-3 fatty acids is increased."

Researchers at the University of Kansas Medical Center in Kansas City reported in the *Journal of the American College of Nutrition* (10:220–227, 1991) that long-term treatment of hyperlipidemic patients with fish oil reduces triglyceride levels. However, blood levels of cholesterol remained essentially unchanged. During the 6-month study, the volunteers were randomly assigned to take 3, 6, 9 or 12 capsules of fish oil daily. This provided from 1.25 to 5 grams of omega-3 fatty acids.

## INHIBITS CANCER

In a study at the American Health Foundation in Valhalla, New York, the research team concluded that, whereas corn oil increased the risk of colon cancer in this instance, fish oil seemed to inhibit both the development and progression of cancer. The study, reported in *Cancer Research* (51:487–491, 1991), utilized corn oil, since it is rich in omega-6 fatty acids, and fish oil, which, of course contains omega-3 fatty acids.

The researchers found that the corn oil diet increased the incidence and multiplicity of colon adenocarcinomas during the post-initiation stage. The fish oil diet did the opposite, apparently by altering carcinogen metabolism and modifying prostaglandin synthesis, the researchers added.

Prostaglandins, which are hormonelike fats, are essential for our body chemistry, and we must have a supply of unsaturated fats to produce them, reported H. L. Newbold, M.D. in *Dr. Newbold's Type A/Type B Weight Loss Book* (Keats Publishing, New Canaan, Conn. 1991). Prostaglandins help to lower blood pressure, and they provide smooth muscle tissue such as in the intestinal tract and the uterus, he continued.

"An article in the scientific journal *Nature* stated that fish oils decrease blood clotting and increase bleeding time," Dr. Newbold said. "The eating of oily fish may explain the low rate of heart disease in Greenland and among the Eskimos. Cod liver oil is fish oil."

## DECREASED SERUM CHOLESTEROL

In an article in the *Journal of Nutrition* (121:165–169, 1991), researchers at the University of Uppsala in Sweden found that fish oil supplemented with vitamin E decreased serum cholesterol 48 percent and fibrinogen by 11 percent. The latter is a blood-clotting constituent.

The Swedish scientists concluded that the improved cardiac risk with the vitamin E-fish oil combo might be due to the inhibition of fatty acid peroxidation with a reduced formation of malondialdehyde and an increased amount of omega-3 fatty acids available for metabolism. This, they added, would reduce the production of triglycerides and fibrinogen in the liver and perhaps lessen the risk for developing cardiovascular disease.

Whether you are eating deep-water fish, such as herring, salmon, bluefish, tuna, sardines or mackerel or taking fish oil capsules, you are assured of having many health benefits.

# EVENING PRIMROSE OIL

## *Its Amazing Nutrients and the Health Benefits They Can Give You*

RICHARD A. PASSWATER, PH.D

At one time evening primrose was known chiefly for its beauty. A few knew of its healing powers as an herb, but not much attention was paid to this lovely plant.

There are several varieties of the evening primrose, and all are classified in the Onagraceae family (genpus Primula). The most common varieties beautifying North America are Oenothera biennis, Oenothera caespitosa and Oenothera hookeri. Of course, most people would more easily recognize one of the common names such as King's Cure-all, sandlily, rockrose, hooker, sun drop, night willow herb, coffee plant, fever plant, scurvish, scabish, cabish, German ranpion, large ranpion, gumbo primrose, tree primrose, etc.

Perhaps the reason evening primrose has so many common names is that varieties grow throughout North America along streams and roadsides as border plants and in the high deserts as a field plant. It grows from sea level to 9000 feet above sea level.

Jack Challem, author of *What Herbs Are All About* (Keats Publishing, Inc., New Canaan, Conn. 1980), describes the white-tufted evening primrose as a delicately petaled, large-flowered 3" diameter plant with a light-green vein running down the centers of the lance-shaped leaves. Although some varieties are shorter, the plants are generally two to five feet tall. Challem recollects seeing the evening primrose in bloom for the first time. "They looked at first like tissue paper strewn across the desert. I had to stop because it looked like someone had littered the desert. . . ." He adds, "The delicate flowers generally last one night and wither to a pinkish color. They bloom in the evening and are pollinated by night-flying insects."

The white-tufted evening primrose produces flowers ranging from white to bright yellow, while other varieties produce red or lavender blooms. The plants are biennials requiring two years to bloom, after which they die in the fall.

The Pilgrims learned of the medicinal properties of the evening primrose from the Indians. The Indians used whole-plant extracts of the evening primrose externally to heal wounds and soothe skin inflammations and eruptions. They used it internally to control coughs and infections. The evening primrose was quickly exported to England where it soon became known as "King's Cure-all."

Chief Two-Trees of the Cherokee nation, who studied with several medicine men, reported that evening primrose was used to lessen spasms, as a sedative, pain killer, diuretic and a mild astringent. The root is used for making a cough syrup that is especially effective against whooping cough, asthmatic cough and tuberculosis cough. The sedative effect varies with the species and with the person. M. Moore suggests that the sedative effect is due to the potassium nitrate found in all parts of the plant.[1]

The evening primrose today is desired not as an herb, but as the only known substantial source of a nutrient which is the focus of much current research. Scientists have found that the oil of the evening primrose seed is rich in gamma linolenic acid (GLA), a rare nutrient that can help alleviate many health problems ranging from heart disease to arthritis to skin disorders. Research indicates that evening primrose oil may also be effective as part of any program to lose weight or to overcome alcoholism or schizophrenia.

Evening primrose oil is the richest source of GLA as the oil is 9 percent GLA. GLA should not be confused with linoleic acid or the common form of linolenic acid, which is the ineffective alpha-linolenic acid or ALA. GLA is essential to good health because it is needed in order for the body to make a family of hormone-like compounds that control every organ in the body. These compounds especially affect the heart and circulation, skin and defense mechanism against disease. The members of this vital family of compounds are called *prostaglandins* (PGs). Anyone having a deficiency of GLA will also have a shortage of PGs, resulting in impaired health. The nutritional optimization of PG is a revolutionary breakthrough in health care.

Even though your doctor may have prescribed evening primrose oil as a dietary supplement, it is not a drug. It does not force your body to do or make anything. The extra GLA made available in your diet allows your body to make all the PGs needed for health. The roles of evening primrose oil are both that of a nutrient and that of a remedial dietetic.

Evening primrose oil has been used to:

- Lower weight in the overweight without dieting
- Lower blood cholesterol
- Lower blood pressure to normal
- Heal or improve eczema
- Stop rheumatoid arthritis in moderate cases
- Normalize saliva and tear production
- Relieve premenstrual pain
- Slow progression of multiple sclerosis
- Improve acne when taken with zinc
- Improve behavior and function of hyperactive children
- Improve fingernails
- Alleviate hangover

All of the benefits listed above have been documented in humans. Evening primrose oil has also been demonstrated to have the following effects on laboratory animals:

- Slowed rate of growth of breast cancer
- Reduced risk of thrombosis
- Prevention of the development of arthritis

Clinical trials to investigate the effects in humans are planned.

## GLA—A KEY NUTRIENT

GLA (gamma-linolenic acid) has achieved recognition in nutrition only relatively recently. It was previously believed that everyone could make their own GLA from an essential fatty acid called linoleic acid. We have learned that GLA is not being adequately produced by many people, resulting in major health problems.

Essential fatty acids (EFAs) are the simplest compounds that can be used for manufacturing other compounds in the body. EFAs are essential to the diet because they themselves cannot be made in the body. Their importance is that they are used to make other needed compounds, such as prostaglandins and thromboxanes. EFAs are useless, however, unless they can be converted to other compounds.

While it is true that all essential fatty acids are polyunsaturated fatty acids, not many polyunsaturated fatty acids are essential to the diet. In fact, scientists believe that *only* linoleic acid is a dietary essential. The body can make other vital fatty acids as needed provided it is well-nourished with vitamins and minerals.

EFAs are very much like vitamins. The absence of EFAs causes deficiency diseases, just as a vitamin deficiency would. Before the EFAs were isolated and identified as fatty acids, they were actually thought to be vitamins by researchers. Collectively the EFAs were referred to as "vitamin F" during the early phases of research (the term is obsolete now).

The symptoms noted in animals deficient in EFA include:

- Hair loss
- Painful, swollen joints
- Dry, scaly skin
- Irritability
- Lethargy
- Infertility
- Infections
- Liver problems
- Poor tissue structure

These symptoms appear in humans as well, but few physicians think in terms of EFA deficiency; after all, we eat too much fat and food tables tell us that the "average person" consumes more than enough EFA. Only recently have studies demonstrated that factors in the typical diet could block GLA formation in the body. It is the GLA and the resulting prostaglandins (PGs) that are important to health. EFA is just a starting point.

Another problem is that many people are deficient in the vitamins and minerals needed to finish the job of GLA and PG production. The above symptoms of EFA deficiency are similar to those of vitamin B6 deficiency and aging, both of which effect the production of GLA. Let's look at this more closely.

We can make GLA in our bodies out of the essential fatty acid *cis*-linoleic acid—provided that the reaction is not blocked by *trans*-linoleic acid. Cis- and trans- refer to the arrangement of the atoms in EFA compounds. The transformation of EFAs to GLA may also be blocked by deficiencies of vitamin B6, zinc, magnesium or insulin. We *can* make GLA in our bodies, but the question is can we make enough GLA fast enough for optimum health? The answer for many people is "no" due to genetic limitations, nutrient deficiencies or blockage by other dietary factors.

So many people must depend on their diets to get optimal amounts of GLA. Evening primrose oil is an ideal way of obtaining GLA for two reasons: It is rich in GLA, and it is free of blocking agents.

There is a great biological difference caused by the very small structural difference between cis- and trans- forms of fatty acids. Trans-fatty acids differ from the naturally occurring cis-fatty acids in the manner in which they become incorporated into membranes of cells, thus affecting their function.[2] Trans-fatty acids are also incorporated differently into triglycerides and phospholipids. More importantly, trans-fatty acids greatly affect the utilization of EFA; trans-linoleic acid (tLA) blocks the utilization of cis-linoleic acid (cLA). The presence of trans-fatty acids in the diet increases the EFA requirement and aggravates the symptoms of EFA deficiency.[3]

The cis- form occurs naturally, while, with few exceptions, the trans- form is manufactured by man. Trans-fatty acids are widely distributed in the diet because processed vegetable oils are used in a vast variety of foods. Vegetable oils contain generous amounts of cis-polyunsaturated fatty acids. However, commercial processing designed to improve stability and odor converts a substantial amount of the cis-polyunsaturated fatty acids to trans-polyunsaturated fatty acid. When vegetable or seed oils are hydrogenated to improve consistency and stability in producing margarine, not only are saturated fatty acids formed, but trans-polyunsaturated fatty acids are produced in great quantity. As an example, stick margarine contains from 25 to 35 percent trans-fatty acids, tub margarine 15 to 25 percent, shortening 20 to 30 percent, and salad oils 0 to 15 percent.[3]

The typical American diet blocks the utilization of cLA. Estimates of biologically active cLA are high because both cLA and tLA are lumped together. A large percentage of the cLA that is in the diet is useless because of the blocking fats or deficiencies in vitamin B6, zinc and magnesium. GLA bypasses these problems. Adding evening primrose oil to the diet is a prudent step.

TABLE 1

IMPORTANT POLYUNSATURATED FATTY ACID CONTENT OF THE MAJOR OILS

| Oil | cis-linoleic (cLA) | gamma-linolenic (GLA) | Blocking Fats |
|---|---|---|---|
| Evening primrose | 73% | 9% | 18% |
| Safflower | 73% | — | 27% |
| Corn | 57% | — | 43% |
| Sunflower | 58% | — | 42% |
| Soybean | 51% | — | 49% |
| Peanut | 29% | — | 71% |
| Olive | 8% | — | 92% |
| Coconut | 2% | — | 98% |

FIGURE 1

GLA AND PG PRODUCTION

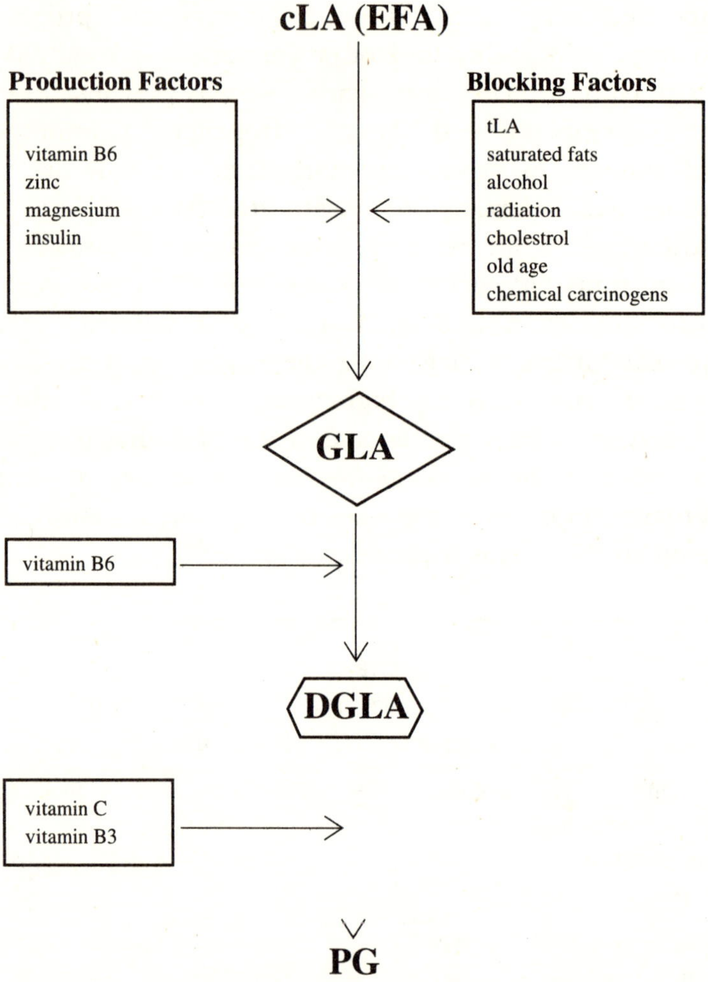


Shown are nutrient deficiencies and blocking factors which interfere with the body's production of GLA which is needed for the production of prostaglandins. PG regulates all organs and cells thus affecting the health of the body in many ways. When cLA is blocked, then you must get your GLA from the diet so that you can make optimal amounts of PG.

## PROSTAGLANDINS—THE HEALTH CONTROLLERS

All of the chemistry presented so far establishes that we need gamma-linolenic acid in the diet. Even though the typical diet contains too much fat, not enough of the essential fatty acid cis-linoleic acid is converted to GLA.

The reason that we need the body well stocked with GLA is so that the body can make as much PG as it needs. The various human PGs are not readily obtainable in the diet. Furthermore, PGs are complex molecules, and are destroyed by the digestive process. Our body's own production of GLA should be fortified to assure optimal levels of PG for the following reasons:

- Because PGs control a multitude of essential functions in the body and are involved in a diverse array of disorders such as heart attacks, high blood pressure, arthritis, menstrual cramps, allergies, asthma, migraine headaches, fertility, glaucoma and, perhaps, cancer.
- Because PGs are not stored. Every tissue makes PG as needed. The effects of PGs are very brief because they are quickly inactivated by enzymes. The functional integrity of some organ systems depend on a balance of PGs which act in opposite ways.

Scientists have learned of the functions of approximately twenty different PGs. Of them, those of the families designated as E family and F family are the most important. They are abbreviated for convenience as PGE and PGF. One other PG family is of particular interest, that of the 'I' family. One member of the PGI family, $PGI_2$, often called "prostacyclin," is a particularly potent cellular regulator and anti-clotting agent. The most interesting family, though, is PGE, and the most marvelous member of this family is $PGE_1$.

The subscripts refer to the EFA used as the starting point in its production. The PG series made from GLA are designated by the subscript 1. The PG series made from arachidonic acid (AA) are designated by the subscript 2, and the series from eicosapentaenoic acid (EPA) by the subscript 3. The biological differences between the three series seem to be dependent solely on the differences in the number of double bonds in the precursor polyunsaturated fatty acid.

It seems that PGs made from GLA and EPA have desirable functions that are often held in check by PGs from AA. $PGE_1$ and $PGE_3$ are protective against heart attacks caused by blood clot. $PGE_1$, $PGE_3$ and $PGI_2$ keep the blood platelets from sticking together, but $PGE_2$ promotes platelet aggregation (the first step in clotting).[4] A balance of $PGE_1$ and $PGE_3$ versus $PGE_2$ thus maintains the proper clotting mechanism. However, a shortage of $PGE_1$ or $PGE_3$ or an excess of $PGE_2$ will increase the tendency to form heart attack-causing blood clots in the coronary arteries.

A *balance* of the appropriate fatty acids in the diet is required to maintain a proper clotting mechanism. Unfortunately, many people eat too much AA and tLA and not enough GLA, cLA and EPA.

In general, PGs of the E family and F family produce contrasting effects; and in some instances $PGE_1$ and $PGE_2$ have opposing actions.[5] $PGE_1$ is an effective inhibitor of blood clotting, while $PGE_2$ accelerates blood clotting.[6] $PGE_1$ has a diuretic action, whereas $PGE_2$ causes the kidneys to retain salt, thereby increasing water retention. Thus, $PGE_2$ has been implicated as a possible factor in high blood pressure.[7]

Dr. David Horrobin of the Institute for Innovative Medicine in Montreal, a foremost researcher in the relationships between cLA, GLA and PG production, stated: "The level of $PGE_1$ is of crucial importance to the body. A fall in the level of $PGE_1$ will lead to a potentially catastrophic series of untoward consequences including increased vascular reactivity, enhanced [blood clotting], elevated cholesterol production, [diabetic-like changes in insulin release], enhanced risk of auto-immune disease, enhanced release of AA, enhanced risk of inflammatory disorders and susceptibility to depression."[8]

$PGE_1$ is necessary for normal function of the T-cells of the immune system (these cells reject foreign bodies). In cell cultures, $PGE_1$ reduced the rate of cell division in a malignant tissue and restored cell normality. $PGE_1$ reduces the release of inflammation-causing lysosomes, and slows the formation of inflammation-producing $PGE_2$ by blocking AA release from storage. It has prevented arthritis in rats and auto-immune disease in mice.

$PGE_1$ affects the release of compounds from nerve cells that transmit nerve impulses; it also seems to regulate calcium movement in cells.

$PGE_1$ has many more functions that affect several disease processes, as described below.

## HEART DISEASE AND EVENING PRIMROSE OIL

What relationship could this ubiquitous delicate flower, the evening primrose, have to a healthy heart? The relationship is not esoteric, rather it concerns a nutrient found in the seed of the evening primrose that is widely required to restore a physiological balance that ensures heart health.

Most Western diets today have two flaws: 1.) Diets are deficient in some nutrients and 2.) the diet has too many superfluous nutrients. Modern Western diets have insufficient quantities of the essential fatty acid (EFA) cis-linoleic acid (cLA) and certain vitamins (including vitamins B6, C and E) and minerals (including magnesium and selenium). Typical diets also contain fats, called trans-fats, that block the utilization of cLA. These dietary flaws hamper the production of prostaglandins, required for heart and circulatory system health.

### HEART ATTACKS

Heart attacks are caused by insufficient blood reaching the heart or a serious irregularity in the heart beat. The problem of insufficient blood can be caused by clots in a coronary artery, resulting in blocked blood flow, or by spasms in an artery. Fat and cholesterol-containing deposits contribute to clot formation.

When blood supply through a coronary artery is insufficient, the tissue fed by that artery dies. If the area of destroyed heart tissue is small, the damage is not serious and tough fibrous scar tissue forms over the damaged region. Recovery can be complete.

The formation of a clot or an occlusion in a coronary artery is called "coronary thrombosis" and the resultant death of heart tissue is called "myocardial infarction."

## PREVENTION OF OCCLUSION-BASED HEART ATTACKS

Blood is normally a slippery fluid. If we were to cut ourselves, however, all of our blood could run out unless something would plug the wound. The body does this by causing the blood to clot. Under the conditions of a wound, blood platelets (plate-shaped components in blood about one-half the size of red blood cells) adhere together to initiate the clotting procedure.

The tendency for blood to clot is measured by an index called the "platelet adhesion index." A healthy person would typically have a platelet adhesion index near 20. This means that their blood is not sticky. The measurement is made by flowing blood over glass beads in an instrument. The number 20 indicates that 20 percent of the platelets stuck to the beads. Measurements taken of recent heart attack victims are as high as 90, indicating that the blood is highly prone to clotting.

Normally, artery walls make prostacyclin ($PGI_2$) a substance that prevents the platelets from sticking to each other or to artery walls. However, arteries damaged by fat and cholesterol deposits, high blood pressure, or injury do not make adequate amounts of $PGI_2$. Platelet adhesion to cholesterol deposits results in rapid buildup of a clot, which can impede blood flow.

As we have seen, $PGE_1$ and $PGE_3$ can both reduce blood platelet adhesion. The dietary intake of GLA in evening primrose oil is an important aid in keeping blood slippery and preventing clotting. Vitamin E and fish oils (EPA) also aid in restoring proper blood slipperiness.

Thus, cholesterol deposits may be present in arteries, but this condition does not dictate the occurrence of a heart attack. Coronaries were unknown until the turn of the century, when food processing began refining vitamins B6 and E and the mineral magnesium out of the food supply. Heart attacks became epidemic after 1920 when man-made trans-fats which block cLA utilization were introduced to the food supply. The main problem is not the deposits per se, but sticky blood. Evening primrose oil bypasses this problem by providing GLA and making $PGE_1$, which keeps blood slippery.

## PREVENTING SPASM-TYPE HEART ATTACKS

There is a case when normal blood slipperiness will not provide enough protection. Let's consider artery construction for a moment to see why.

Arteries have a built-in defense mechanism against a very strong shock. The artery walls can constrict tightly to shut off blood flow if they are cut during severe injury. However, sometimes the artery walls are stimulated to contract by emotional shock or stress. Artery spasms are more apt to occur in conjunction with dietary imbalances such as magnesium deficiency or available cLA deficiency.

Spasm-type heart attacks were thought to be rare a few years ago. An Italian research team found that at least 20 percent of all fatal heart attacks were artery spasms. New testing techniques were developed that indicate that a larger percentage—perhaps the majority—of fatal heart attacks are caused by artery spasms.

Artery spasms are usually fatal only when the constricting artery is already partially blocked by cholesterol and fat deposits. Of course, what started investigators into this direction of research were the heart attacks observed in young people with deposit-free arteries.

The mechanism involved in spasm-type heart attack is well established. Stress causes the nerves to release chemicals which in turn cause the arteries to constrict. The reduced blood supply also reduces the oxygen available to the artery muscle. If this oxygen reduction is mild, the artery relaxes. However, if the oxygen supply is severely reduced, the muscle goes into spasms.

Keep in mind that cigarette smokers already have reduced available oxygen, and smokers have greater risk for the spasm to develop rather than artery relaxation. Stress and smoking are a killing combination.

During artery spasm, $PGI_2$ is not released and $PGE_2$ may be released. As a result blood platelets clump together and adhere to the artery wall to form a more lasting seal. This is a key point. It takes two to three hours for permanent heart tissue change to occur. The heart tissue will not die if the blood shortage is only temporary. If the artery spasm can be relaxed in a short time, no permanent damage will occur. However, if the spasm lasts sufficiently long, a blood clot occurs which makes a seal lasting long enough to cause tissue death.

## OTHER HEART PROBLEMS ARE RELATED

The partially blocked artery increases the probability of heart damage by either clot formation or arterial spasm. If the area of the heart affected is the "pacemaker" region controlling heart beat, an irregularity may result in a beat that is too weak to pump blood. This grossly irregular beat is called ventricular fibrillation. Ventricular fibrillation can have other causes besides infarction (tissue death).

Angina pectoris is the severe chest pain that develops during exertion or stress. The partially clogged arteries can supply sufficient blood to meet heart oxygen needs only when the person is resting. Movement or emotional stress creates a greater oxygen demand which cannot be met. The result is that the heart releases chemicals that cause pain and warn the person to slow down. A continued oxygen shortage can lead to artery spasm and then tissue damage.

Dilation of the coronary arteries increases blood flow thus quenching the pain. Nitroglycerin dilates arteries, and so does $PGE_1$. Many have found that increased dietary GLA reduces their need for nitroglycerin and can greatly reduce the number and severity of their angina attacks.

Evening primrose oil has a lot to offer the heart patient. However, it is not a drug and it doesn't work immediately during a heart attack. Evening primrose oil does offer the angina patient partial relief in a relatively short time, however.[9]

Typical effective supplement protocol for heart disease that has also lowered blood cholesterol and helped normalize body weight has been three to four 500 milligram evening primrose oil capsules in the morning with an equal amount taken in the evening.[10]

Vitamin E should also be considered for use in a strategy against heart disease. Vitamin E increases the formation of prostacyclin ($PGI_2$), thus lowering blood platelet adhesion. There are also reports that vitamin E increases the "good" cholesterol carrier, called high density lipoprotein (HDL), that is protective against heart disease.

## ARTHRITIS

Arthritis lessens the quality of life for millions of people. Often the pain of arthritis can be controlled, but the damage to the bone joint continues until mobility is lost. There are two common types of arthritis: rheumatoid arthritis and osteoarthritis. Evening primrose oil has been shown to be effective against rheumatoid arthritis; at this writing it has not been tried against osteoarthritis, a "wear and tear" type of damage.

Rheumatoid arthritis begins as an inflammation in the membrane that produces the fluid that lubricates bone joints. This membrane is called the synovial membrane. The cause of the inflammation is not certain, but many medical researchers believe that the body's immune system mistakenly attacks the joints, thereby causing inflammation. Diet and stress have also been suggested as being responsible for

EVENING PRIMROSE OIL AND BLOOD CHOLESTEROL LEVELS

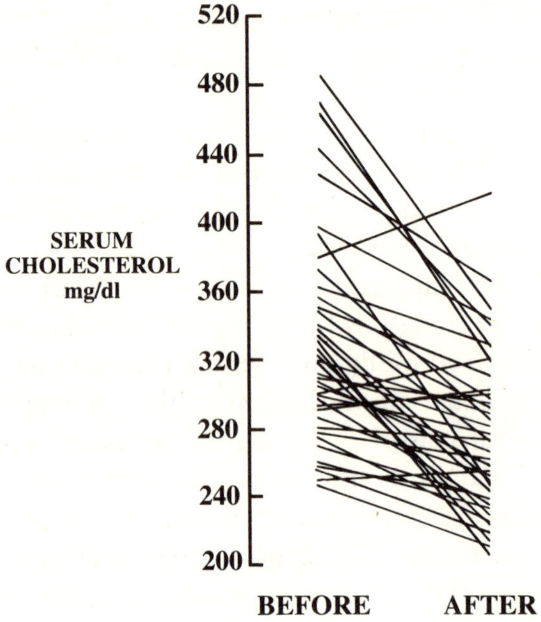


Changes in blood cholesterol levels in individuals who took four to six capsules of evening primrose oil for periods of two to twelve months.

initiating the inflammation, and it's possible that all three are involved. Perhaps one causes arthritis in some people, while another is the cause in others. It's even possible that all three must be involved in the same person to initiate the inflammation.

When the synovial membrane becomes inflamed, the blood supply to the membrane increases, white blood cells gather in the membrane, and swelling occurs. The swelling can become severe enough to push the bones apart. The inflammation causes the synovial membrane to release chemicals called lysosomal enzymes that destroy cartilage and bone. The body tries to repair this damage but usually forms irregular patches and rough bumps. These outgrowths aggravate the problem and decrease joint function.

The inflammation is brought about by the 2 series prostaglandins produced from arachidonic acid (AA). The inflammation can be reduced by slowing down the release of stored AA or slowing the production of $PGE_2$.

It is becoming clear that there is an interrelationship between PG, vitamin E, aspirin and steroid drugs. The interrelationship can be explained by looking at the pathways for using EFA. So far we have concentrated on how EFA is made into PG. However, there is another important pathway wherein EFA produces particularly noxious compounds called "*leukotrienes.*" Leukotrienes do have a positive function. They are desirable during wound healing. However, they can be released under other conditions that can be bothersome.

Poorly controlled leukotriene production is suspected of causing such unpleasant effects as arthritic inflammation and the painful breast lumps of cystic mastitis. Leukotrienes are formed from arachidonic acid (AA). AA can be converted to PG or leukotriene. Excesses of either $PGE_2$ or leukotriene can be a problem. $PGE_2$ can lead to unwanted blood clotting, pain or fever depending on the tissues in which it is produced. Aspirin can reduce the production of $PGE_2$. This explains how aspirin reduces pain and fever, and how it can under certain conditions reduce the risk of a clot forming in the coronary artery. This also explains how aspirin has the undesirable side effects of gastrointestinal bleeding. It also explains why aspirin reduces the pain of arthritis with little effect on inflammation.

Dr. David Cornwell of Ohio State has elucidated the mechanism of leukotriene production. Leukotriene production can be brought under control by slowing the release of AA from storage or by slowing the conversion of AA to leukotriene with vitamin E.

Drugs such as corticosteroids or indomethacin act on pain and inflammation by slowing AA release from storage. Thus both $PGE_2$ and leukotriene production are slowed, which in turn controls both pain and inflammation. Unfortunately, these drugs also have serious drawbacks. Neither aspirin nor steroids affect the long term course of arthritis because they block the production of the desirable $PGE_1$. However, there is an alternative method to slow AA release from storage.

The preferred way to control AA release from storage is by $PGE_1$

manipulation. If adequate GLA is available, then $PGE_1$ can be produced to balance $PGE_2$ and also control AA release. It is always preferable to utilize natural body compounds to regulate the body rather than to use synthetic drugs, such as aspirin or indomethacin, if the same degree of control can be achieved.

Fairly strong evidence exists that in some individuals the inflammation is caused or at least aggravated by food allergies. Foods of the nightshade family (including potatoes, tomatoes, peppers, paprika and eggplant) and wheat are particularly suspect for such food allergies.

If you are interested in checking to see if you are the victim of food allergy, you could consider the merits of eliminating the potential offenders from your diet for three months. You might wish to first remove all nightshade plants, and if that doesn't help, add them back and then remove all wheat products.

Dr. David Horrobin of Montreal explains that in some patients such a nutritional approach alone may be adequate, while in others, additional support from drugs may be necessary.[11]

Evening primrose oil is effective in controlling rheumatoid arthritis in a substantial number of patients.[12] However, three factors should be noted. First, evening primrose oil does not benefit patients receiving more than trivial doses of steroids, indomethacin-like or aspirin-like drugs. This is because they have conflicting action on $PGE_1$. However, evening primrose oil can be taken and then the drug dosage reduced after one to three months.

Second, the benefits of evening primrose oil do not become apparent for one to three months. Some patients experience a specific transient setback during the first week or two, although they do well in the long run.

Third, there is preliminary evidence that the disease may be actually *halted* in some patients, as opposed to the action of the drugs.[11] Of course, it would be too much to expect reversal of pre-existing damage.

Evening primrose oil has been helpful in many patients at the three to four gram level of intake per day. This represents three to four

500 milligram capsules taken at both morning and evening. Other dietary deficiencies should be corrected. This is especially true of vitamins B6, C, E and pantothenic acid.

## WEIGHT CONTROL

Some overweight people eat more food than normal weight people. On the other hand a great many fat people eat no more—and even less—than thin people. "But I eat like a bird" is often exclaimed by the frustrated perennial dieter. Of course, if you eat more calories than you burn, you will put on fat. However, the key is that some people do not burn their calories as easily as others.

In the past, this difference has been explained as being due to differences in basal metabolism (the energy needed just to keep the body alive). This basic energy-burning rate is dependent on genetics, exercise level and hormonal relationships. We are now aware of a separate mechanism that burns calories and helps determine who's thin and who's fat.

Thin people seem to have a well-functioning mechanism to burn off extra calories, whereas fat people have a faulty mechanism—or the mechanism is poorly developed. The body has a special tissue of brown fat located in the back of the neck and along the backbone. The brown coloration is due to the high concentration of cellular energy-producing (fat burning) units called mitochondria. The brown fat burns calories not to produce energy for body movement, but solely for heat. One role of brown fat is weight stabilization, another is adaptation to cold weather.

Appetite control is centered in a region of the brain called the ventromedial hypothalamus. Appetite regulation utilizes a feedback mechanism that senses insulin and amino acid content of the blood. It is believed that the ventromedial hypothalamus can switch on the brown fat tissue whenever excess calories are consumed. Obese persons may either have a faulty "switch" or they may have insufficient amounts of brown fat.

Before the brown fat mechanism was elucidated, many investigators were seeking the "mechanism X". It was obvious that an unknown mechanism existed, but the mechanism was so different from what was expected that it was overlooked. The role of brown fat in weight regulation was more or less uncovered by research into cold adaptation.

The "brown fat" discovery was made by several researchers including Dr. David G. Nicholls of the University of Dundee, Scotland; Dr. Jean Himms-Hagen of the University of Ottawa; Dr. Michael Stock of St. George's Hospital medical school in London; and Dr. George Bray of the University of California at Los Angeles.

The gamma-linolenic acid (GLA) content of evening primrose oil has a stimulating effect on brown fat tissue. GLA forms certain prostaglandins that accelerate the mitochondria activity in the brown fat.

A large clinical trial in Heidelberg, West Germany, demonstrated that heavier people had less polyunsaturated fatty acids and conversely[13] thinner individuals had a higher proportion. Those with high polyunsaturated fatty acid content tended to be of normal weight. Dr. David Horrobin of Montreal postulates that fat people may be suffering from a polyunsaturated fatty acid deficiency. Dr. Horrobin has found that GLA is remarkably effective in causing weight loss, and that evening primrose oil is a particularly valuable dietary component in those who want to lose weight.[14]

In a study by Dr. K.S. Vaddadi and Dr. David Horrobin, evening primrose oil lowered body weight in about half of those who were more than 10 percent overweight. *The effect was achieved without conscious dieting,* although those who lost weight reported that they spontaneously felt less hungry.[14]

Keep in mind that body fat is also determined by what you eat and when you eat, as well as how much you eat. Good quality foods produce less body fat than junk foods because of their effect on insulin release.[15]

Never try to crash diet. The results are short term. Adjust your eating behavior to good nutritional foods, spaced into frequent small meals, prior to your energy needs. Lose a pound or two a week and you have a better chance to keep it off.

EVENING PRIMROSE OIL AND WEIGHT NORMALIZATION

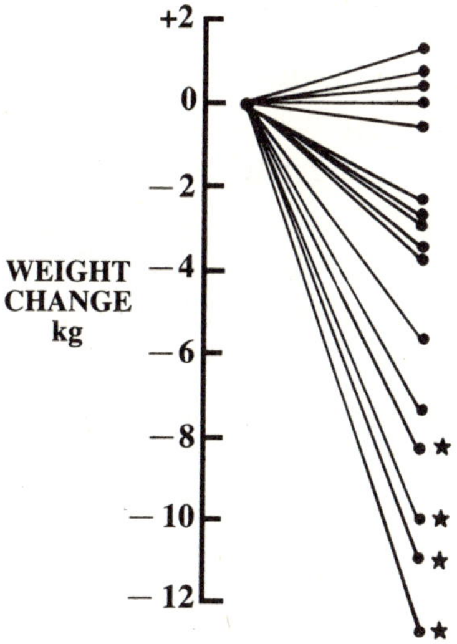


Changes in weight in 16 individuals who exceeded their ideal body weight by more than 10 percent took evening primrose oil for 6 to 8 weeks. The starred individuals took eight capsules per day while the others took four capsules per day. No weight changes occurred in 22 individuals who were within 10 percent of their ideal body weight. (*courtesy of Dr. David Horrobin*)

Balance your diet and take a vitamin and mineral supplement to ensure that you maintain adequate nourishment even though your food quality may be reduced.

Consider the beneficial effect of evening primrose oil on brown fat tissue and weight normalization.

## CANCER AND IMMUNITY

It is now known that what you eat helps your body fight off cancer. Deficiencies of any of the major antioxidant nutrients (vitamins A, C and E plus the mineral selenium) have been shown to increase susceptibility to cancer in man and other animals.[16,17] Dietary supplements of these same antioxidant nutrients have been shown to increase resistance to cancer.

Several biochemical mechanisms are involved in the protective roles of the antioxidant nutrients, but the most important is the stimulation of the immune response. Now we have learned that we have a new ally in our natural defense against cancer. The hormone-like PGs affect the immune system. One PG, made from the gamma-linolenic acid found in evening primrose oil, stimulates the T-cells of the immune system and amazingly, *reverts cancer cells back to normal cells in test tube experiments.*

This compound, called PGE, has been extensively discussed throughout this chapter. $PGE_1$ is required for the T-cells (T-lymphocytes) of the immune system to attack a cancer. In fact, $PGE_1$ plays a major role in the regulation of thymus gland development, as well as in T-cell function. T-cells play a critical role in cellular immunity. A deficiency in GLA, vitamin C, vitamin B6 or zinc leads to inadequate $PGE_1$ production and thus defective T-cell function.[18]

Thus, these nutrients are required in optimal quantities to maintain optimal immunity.

The immune system is our last line of defense against cancer. Our first line of defense is our liver which can detoxify cancer-causing chemicals. Our second line of defense is the cell membrane which controls cell nourishment and protects cells against invasion by cancer-causing chemicals.

Many scientists believe that healthy people routinely develop precancerous cells that are destroyed by the immune system before they can form a full-fledged cancer. Strengthening of the immune system to prevent—and perhaps overcome—cancer is not a new strategy. However, reversing cancer cells back to normal cells is a new approach to cancer treatment.

Dr. David Horrobin writes in *Medical Hypotheses* (1979):

> Cancer therapy is dominated by the idea that treatment must aim at destruction of cancer cells. The goal is to exploit

> some difference between the cancer cells and the normal cells which will allow the cancerous ones to be selectively destroyed. The selectivity of current chemotherapy and radiation therapy, such as it is, depends on the idea that the already damaged regulatory functions of cancer cells can be totally disrupted more easily than those of normal cells. Since the purpose of these treatments is to produce damage, it is not surprising that they harm normal cells. It is thus not surprising that most cancer therapeutic agents are themselves carcinogens and vice versa. A more rational aim in cancer would be the normalization of cancer cells by techniques which will do no harm to normal tissues. I propose that we already have the necessary information to enable this to be carried out.
>
> Very little attention has been paid to the possibility of normalizing cancer cells. This is largely because the dominant theme of research into the cause of cancer is that the disease is brought about by irreversible and uncontrollable mutation, probably within the nuclear DNA or possibly within one of the other nucleic acid pools such as that in the mitochondria. However, it is by no means clear that carcinogenic mutations can never be repaired, nor that irreversible mutations are necessarily uncontrollable, nor that mutation is always a necessary condition of cancer development. Indeed, several lines of evidence indicate that the idea of treating cancer by normalizing cancer cells is not completely unrealistic.[18]

Cancer cells are already defective and have a high rate of death. The cancer grows only because the proliferation rate exceeds the cell death rate. If proliferation can be controlled by normalizing cell function, then the already damaged cancer cells will die and the cancer will regress.

$PGE_1$ is one of the most potent natural agents which is believed to induce cancer cell reversal.[19] Even genetic mutations can be kept in check and sometimes reversed by $PGE_1$.

Cancer cells produce excessive amounts of the 2 series PG and cannot make $PGE_1$.[18] Now there is evidence that $PGE_1$ together with thromboxane ($TX_2$), another important family of compounds made from cLA, AA and EPA, can reverse all the abnormalities common to cancer cells.

Dr. Horrobin has proposed that the critical step in cancer cell formation is the loss of the ability to make $PGE_1$ and/or $TX_2$. He believes that restoration of normal $PGE_1$ levels by providing GLA will be of value in reversing cancer growth.

In test tubes or cell cultures, human cells can be transformed to cancer cells by radiation or carcinogens. In the transformation process, the cells lose their ability to convert cLA into GLA, and hence to make $PGE_1$.[18,20,21] The malignant cells can be made normal by exposing them to $PGE_1$.[18,22,23]

The action of vitamin C might be enhanced by administering it with evening primrose oil which would restore the responsiveness of the cells to vitamin C. Trials of the value of combined treatment with vitamin C and evening primrose oil are now in progress at several centers.

## PREMENSTRUAL PAIN, CYSTIC MASTITIS AND BRITTLE NAILS

Evening primrose oil corrects several problems of special interest to women. This may make evening primrose oil the best discovery of the century.

The pain of premenstrual tension is both physical and mental. Increased water retention causes swelling tissues which results in abdominal pain and depression. Depression and irritability result from the brain swelling against the confinement of the skull.

The gradual increase in fluid can produce pain and mood change beginning from two to fourteen days before menstruation starts. Diuretics help reduce the build-up and bring some relief. However, care must be taken to assure an adequate intake of potassium and magnesium, which have a greater rate of loss from the body with the use of diuretics.

It is possible to increase the effectiveness of the relief naturally without the need for diuretics.

Vitamin B6 has been very effective in about 70 percent of the women with premenstrual tension. Also vitamin E has helped many. The interactions of vitamin B6, vitamin E, gamma-linolenic acid (GLA) and prostaglandins (PG) are now understood. Vitamin B6 is needed for the conversion of cis-linoleic acid to the prostaglandin $PGE_1$. Vitamin E helps keep the noxious compounds called leukotrienes from being formed and encourages the production of the preferred $PGE_1$. GLA bypasses the problem of inefficient cis-linoleic acid conversion and also enhances $PGE_1$ production.

British studies have now found that evening primrose oil, the natural source of GLA, can relieve about 90 to 95 percent of women's premenstrual tension.[24] They have found that evening primrose oil alleviates symptoms of two-thirds of the women not helped by anything else, while another 20 percent were greatly improved.

The secret is not to wait until the discomfort begins but to take vitamin B6 and evening primrose oil daily. Many have found that 50 milligrams of vitamin B6 and six 500 milligram capsules of evening primrose oil daily are effective. The evening primrose oil capsules should be divided into two or three doses during the day. Extremely difficult cases may need a total of eight 500 milligram capsules of evening primrose oil and up to 200 milligrams of vitamin B6. Vitamin E is generally helpful in the 100 to 600 milligram range.

Evening primrose oil has also aided women with heavy and prolonged bleeding. Instead of a heavy blood loss for seven to ten days, their periods were reduced to four or five days duration at normal blood loss.

The same protective regimen used for premenstrual tension would be effective for many women with heavy and prolonged periods. Relief should occur within two or three cycles. However, some cases will not respond and surgery to remove the fibroids may be required to relieve the problem.

The most common breast disease is cystic mastitis (also called benign breast disease, fibrocystic disease of the breast, mammary dysplasia, or fibrous mastopathy) which affects about 20 percent of premenopausal women. Lumps or cysts may be tender and painful especially prior to menstrual flow, but the majority of cysts are not painful.

The cause of the cysts is thought to be an overproduction of the hormone prolactin, combined with a shortage of $PGE_1$. Evening primrose oil helps prevent cyst development and speedily removes existing lumps. This was discovered by accident while evening primrose oil was being administered to large numbers of women for other reasons. The disappearance or softening of cysts occurred within a two- to four-month period.

Vitamin E also helps this condition, as we saw in our discussion of the interrelationship of vitamin E and GLA. A "double-blind" study led by Dr. Robert S. London at the Johns Hopkins University School of Medicine and Sinai Hospital in Baltimore found that 85 percent of women with advanced cases of the disease responded within eight weeks to 600 milligrams of vitamin E daily. Forty percent of the women had a *complete disappearance* of the lumps.

The same regimen of evening primrose oil, vitamin B6 and vitamin E, which is effective against premenstrual stress and heavy and prolonged bleeding, appears promising against cystic mastitis. Six to eight 500 milligram capsules of evening primrose oil daily should, by itself, be effective for the vast majority of women. Stubborn cases may need the assist from the other vitamins.

Another surprising result of the research with evening primrose oil is that brittle fingernails harden within about two to six weeks. This response is so consistent that it can be concluded that brittle nails are a newly recognized sign of essential fatty acid deficiency in humans. These findings have been published in the May 1981 issue of the *British Journal of Dermatology*. The benefit of this discovery is obvious to women, but also think about its potential use by doctors to diagnose essential fatty acid deficiency.

## OTHER DISEASES

Other diseases are also responding to evening primrose oil supplementation according to preliminary clinical results. Diseases as diverse as diabetes, alcoholism, schizophrenia, multiple sclerosis, hyperactivity, infertility and eczema are among the many helped by evening primrose oil. Although these diseases do not seem to be related in any way, they all involve a disturbance in prostaglandin balance. The gamma-linolenic acid naturally found in evening primrose oil helps to restore the desired PG balance.

### DIABETES

No definitive studies have been completed on evening primrose oil and diabetes. However, a five-year study led by Dr. A. Houtsmuller found that diabetics on a diet rich in essential fatty acid had significantly less eye and heart disease than those with diets low in the oil.[25]

The roles of PG and insulin are interrelated to the mineral zinc. PG helps zinc absorption and zinc aids the production of 1 series PG.[26] $PGE_1$ is able to enhance various actions of insulin. It is possible that some of the insulin resistance which occurs in diabetes could be due to insufficient $PGE_1$.

### ALCOHOLISM

Alcoholics tend to have elevated $PGE_1$ levels while drinking and then crash to a very low $PGE_1$ level afterwards. This results in the "hangover" syndrome. (Although this is of little or no interest to health-minded readers, you may have friends that would be delighted to know that evening primrose oil cures hangovers.)

$PGE_1$ affects calcium release which in turn affects nerve transmissions. There are many similarities between the "feminized" state of the chronic male alcoholic and men with chronic zinc or essential fatty acid deficiency. There are similarities between the congenital abnormalities associated with zinc deficiency and with the fetal alcohol syndrome. Part of the effect may be due to alcohol depletion of zinc, but another part may be that both lead to failure of normal $PGE_1$ production.[27,28] Thus there is an indication that $PGE_1$ may be a key determinant of mood and that some people may drink alcohol as a means of normalizing their brain level of $PGE_1$. If this is correct, then normalizing their $PGE_1$ level by nutritional means should reduce their craving for alcohol.

## SCHIZOPHRENIA

Schizophrenia is a biochemical disease in which thought processes become disordered. Schizophrenics do not have a "dual personality" or "split mind" as is so commonly believed. If the biochemistry of the collective nerve activity can be normalized, then functional normality resumes.

In 1975, researchers at Guy Hospital in London found that blood platelets from schizophrenics completely failed to produce $PGE_1$. There is reason to believe that normalization of $PGE_1$ production can help schizophrenia.

There may indeed be several "causes" of schizophrenia, but these "causes" may only be different agitators of the real cause—abnormal $PGE_1$ production.

As Dr. David Horrobin wrote in *The Lancet*:

> In recent years it has been suggested that the biological defect in schizophrenia may be related to excess dopamine (a compound involved in nerve transmission) activity, to production of an abnormal opioid or a normal opioid in excess, to a prostaglandin deficiency, to a hypersensitivity to wheat proteins, to an allergic phenomenon, to a defect in zinc metabolism, or to a pineal deficiency. . . . The various concepts are not mutually exclusive, but represent different aspects of the same problem. The final common path in schizophrenia may

be a failure of formation and action of prostaglandins of the 1 series.[29]

Striking case histories have been reported in the medical literature. Dr. K. S. Vaddadi, Senior Registrar in Adult Psychiatry at Bootham Park Hospital in York, England reports the following:

"We have administered evening primrose oil together with penicillin to six severe chronic schizophrenics inadequately controlled by phenothiazines. In all cases, all other drug therapy was withdrawn. No patient has become worse during a 16-week period and in some the improvement has been striking."[30]

Patients who had been severely ill from twelve to twenty-one years in spite of treatment with several different drugs showed a dramatic improvement when oral penicillin was administered in combination with evening primrose oil. (Penicillin is used because it stimulates $PGE_1$ production.)

## MULTIPLE SCLEROSIS

*The Multiple Sclerosis Diet Book* by Dr. Roy Swank touts the virtue of polyunsaturated fatty acids in controlling multiple sclerosis. The diet is controversial, but many other physicians are finding it beneficial.

Polyunsaturated fatty acids are not the main factor. PG formation from the essential fatty acid is the main factor. Better results could possibly come from adding the factors needed to convert cis-linolenic acid to the diet to make GLA, and by removing factors that block GLA formation.

Another approach is to supplement the diet with GLA from evening primrose oil. There are about 3,000 MS patients taking evening primrose oil with good results.[31]

Research with laboratory animals preceded this development. In rats, there is a disease called experimental allergic encephalomyelitis which in some respects is very similar to human MS. Evening primrose oil has been found highly effective in preventing this disease.

As a result of these several studies, patients with MS have begun to take evening primrose oil. The indications are that perhaps 15 to 20 percent of patients may be helped in a major way and another 15 to 20 percent in a minor way; 60 to 70 percent of patients are not helped and in no way is this a cure for the disease. However, in some patients, the improvements have been dramatic and it seems worthwhile to give the oil a trial in all patients. A suitable regime is to start with four capsules per day for three months, to increase this to eight capsules per day for a further three months and to twelve capsules per day for a further three months. If, after this time, there has been no improvement it is probably not worth continuing.

In England, a patients organization called Action for Research on Multiple Sclerosis has accumulated evidence to suggest that evening primrose oil slows down the progression of the disease.

## HYPERACTIVITY

A British group, Hyperactive Children's Support Group (HCSG), assembled information that led them to suspect that hyperactivity might be linked with a problem with PG. More than seventy branch chapters conducted an extensive survey profiling the characteristics of hyperactive children.

In the late 1970s Dr. David Horrobin designed a therapeutic protocol. The preliminary results were encouraging. Dr. Horrobin said, "Studies have been initiated in several countries on the use of primrose oil in hyperactivity. About twenty children were treated with substantial benefit in about two-thirds of them. Some of the responses were dramatic. In one case, a boy who had been threatened with expulsion from school because of his impossible behavior was put on primrose oil without the knowledge of the school authorities. After two weeks on GLA, the teacher who was unaware of the treatment contacted the parents and said that in thirty years' experience she had never seen such a dramatic and abrupt change for the better in a child's behavior. Some children appear to do equally well no matter whether the oil is given by mouth or by rubbing into the skin. In others there is the distinct impression that skin absorption which will by-pass malabsorption problems may have a better effect."

I asked Dr. Horrobin how his observations fit in with those of Dr. Ben Feingold of the Kaiser Foundation Hospital-Permanente Medical Group in San Francisco. Dr. Horrobin replied:

> Our findings dovetail very nicely. Feingold has described a large number of natural food substances and food additives which may precipitate symptoms in hyperactive children. These include natural salicylates, butylated hydroxytoluene (BHT), butylated hydroxyanisole (BHA), tartrazine and other colouring materials. Such materials do not, however, precipitate symptoms in normal children. The agents described by Feingold are almost all known inhibitors of conversion of EFAs to PGs or are chemically related to such known inhibitors. For other reasons my group investigated one of the worst offenders, tartrazine, in my laboratory some years ago. We found that it was an effective inhibitor of PG formation when EFA levels were very low but had little or no effect when EFA levels were high. This suggests the possibility that in children with normal EFA levels the materials will have no effect. The fact that they do have such dramatic effects in hyperactive children may indicate that in those children the levels of EFAs are unusually low.

The survey had uncovered the following six points that suggested EFA might be involved with hyperactivity:

1. Hyperactive male children in HCSG outnumber females by about 3:1, a ratio which fits with surveys in North America. Male animals require a two- to three-fold higher intake of EFAs than females in order to prevent signs of EFA deficiency. Therefore in any situation in which the supply of EFAs is marginal, males are likely to be affected much more substantially than females.
2. About two-thirds of the children in HCSG appear to experience abnormal thirst. Thirst is one of the key features of EFA deficiency in animals.
3. Studies sponsored by HCSG have found low levels of zinc in the hair

of many of their children. A lack of zinc will reduce formation of GLA from cLA and will block mobilization of DGLA.

4. HCSG has found that eczema, asthma and other features of the atopic state are much more common in hyperactive children than in normal ones. Such problems are associated with defective T-cell function which could be caused by lack of enough PGE.
5. HCSG has found that some of their children react badly to wheat products and/or milk. Both wheat and milk may give rise to opioids in the gut as product of partial digestion. Opioids have the capacity to block PGE formation form DGLA under certain conditions.
6. HCSG has many examples of families in which there is only one hyperactive child while other siblings eating exactly the same diet are normal. It is therefore unlikely that hyperactivity is associated with any obvious deficiency of dietary cLA. Hyperactive children could have a defect in EFA absorption which means that they may require much larger amounts of dietary EFAs than normal. Alternately, they may have a defect preventing them from converting cLA to GLA.

## SKIN, ACNE, AND ECZEMA

Essential fatty acids are needed for healthy skin and hair. An EFA deficiency results in skin lesions, flaking dandruff, brittle nails and thinning hair. Correcting the diet by adding more EFA doesn't always work because the EFA may be blocked by trans-fatty acids or the person may not have adequate vitamins B6 and C, or the minerals magnesium and zinc in the diet. Evening primrose oil bypasses this problem by supplying the immediate PG-precursor GLA.

Evening primrose oil by itself has shown little effect on acne, but when given with zinc, it often produces striking improvement.

Research led by Dr. C.R. Lovell at the Department of Dermatology of the Royal Infirmary in Bristol, England has shown that evening primrose oil significantly improved patients with severe atopic eczema. The double-blind, placebo-controlled clinical trial supported the thesis that an EFA abnormality was involved in the disease.

## DRY EYES AND MOUTH

Sjogren's syndrome (failure of saliva and tear gland function coupled with connective tissue disease) and sicca syndrome (failure of saliva and tear gland function without connective tissue disease) both respond to evening primrose oil supplementation. These disorders can aggravate other body processes. Without adequate saliva, teeth are less cleansed and the gastrointestinal system is strained. Thus, relief of these problems by evening primrose oil may prevent other disorders.

A revolution in health care is unfolding due to our new understanding of the role of nutrition and prostaglandins. What has been discussed in this chapter is only the beginning of this revolution. Evening primrose oil provides us with a vital nutritional compound intermediate in $PGE_1$ production that bypasses many of the problems caused by modern Western diets.

# REFERENCES


1. Moore, M. 1979. *Medicinal Herbs of the West* (74). University of New Mexico Press.
   Additional information can be found in herbalogy texts such as:
      Angier, B. 1978. *Field Guide to Medicinal Plants.* Harrisburg, PA: Stackpole Books
      Coon, Nelson. 1963. *Using Plants for Healing.* 1963. Emmaus. PA: Rodale Press.
      Hutchens, A. R. 1969. *Indian Herbalogy of North America.* Windsor, Ontario: Merco Press.
2. Sgoutas, D. and Kummerow, F. A. 1970. *American Journal of Clinical Nutrition* 23:1111.
3. *Dairy Council Digest* 46:6 (Nov.-Dec. 1975).
4. White, A. *et al.* 1978. *Principles of Biochemistry,* 6th ed. New York: McGraw-Hill, p. 643.
5. Ibid., p. 641.
6. Ibid., p. 643.

7. Ibid., p. 644.
8. Horrobin, D. F. 1980. *Medical Hypotheses* 6:785–800.
9. Bierenbaum, M. L. and Oudhof, J. H. Abstract Book, International Prostaglandin Conference, Washington, D.C., May 1979, p. 10.
10. Horrobin, David F. Private communication
11. Ibid.
12. McCormick, J. N. *et al.* 1977. *The Lancet* 2:508.
13. Oster, P. *et al. Research in Experimental Medicine* (Berlin) 175: 287–291.
14. Vaddadi, K. S. and Horrobin, D. F. 1979. *Journal of Medical Science* 7:52.
15. Passwater, Richard A. 1980. *The Easy No-Flab Diet.* New York: Marek Publishers.
16. Passwater, Richard A. 1978. *Cancer and Its Nutritional Therapies.* New Canaan, CT: Keats Publishing, Inc.
17. Passwater, Richard A. 1980. *Selenium as Food and Medicine.* New Canaan, CT: Keats Publishing, Inc.
18. Horrobin, D. F. *et al.* 1979. *Medical Hypotheses* 5:969–985.
19. Horrobin, D. F. *et al.* 1980. *Medical Hypotheses* 6:469–486.
20. Dunbar, L. M. and Bailey, J. M. 1975. *Journal of Biology and Chemistry* 250:1152–1154.
21. Bailey, J. M. 1977. *Lipid Metabolism in Mammals* (2) New York: Plenum Press.
22. Puck, T. T. 1977. *Proceedings of the National Academy of Science* 74:4491–4495.
23. Johnson, G. S. *et al.* 1975. *Proceedings of the National Academy of Science* 68:425–429.
24. Horrobin, David F. Private communication.
25. Houtsmuller, A. J. *et al.* 1980. *Nutritional Metabolism* 24:105–118.
26. Horrobin, D. F. and Cunnane, S. C. 1980. *Medical Hypotheses* 6:277–296.
27. Horrobin, D. F. and Manku, M. S. 1980. *British Medical Journal* 280:1363–1366.
28. Horrobin, D. F. 1980. *Medical Hypotheses* 6:929–942.
29. Horrobin, D. F. 1979. *The Lancet* 529:531.
30. Vaddadi, K. S. 1979. *Prostaglandins and Medicine* 2:77–80.
31. Horrobin, D. F. Private communication.

# What Fat-Phobic Americans Need To Know: Essential Fats Are Vital For Good Health

*They Can Protect Against Heart Disease, Arthritis, Diabetes, PMS, Hyperactivity; Promote Healthy Skin, Hair, And Nails*

Although Americans have been told over and over to avoid excess dietary fat, we are seldom reminded that there are certain healthful fats that we must have to remain well. These are the essential fatty acids (EFAs) that used to be called vitamin F. And, as the name implies, "essential" means that they are as necessary for good health as vitamins and minerals and must be obtained from diet or supplements, since the body cannot manufacture sufficient amounts of them.

## MOST ACTIVE

The EFAs consist of two series, namely, the omega-6 series derived from linoleic acid, and the omega-3 series derived from linolenic acid. The omega-3 fatty acids, which offer protection from heart disease and other complaints, are found in deep-water fish and cold-climate vegetable oils. The omega-6 fatty acids, of which gamma-linolenic acid (GLA) is the most active, are primarily found in warm-weather vegetable oils, such as walnut, wheat germ, soybean, safflower, sunflower, corn and other oils.

Although virtually all vegetable oils contain omega-6 EFAs, they may also contain from a smidgen to large amounts of omega-3 EFAs. For example, linseed/flaxseed oil is 60 percent omega-3 and 20 percent omega-6. Evening primrose oil, borage oil and black currant seed oil, high in gamma-linolenic acid, contain both omega-3 and omega-6.

"Abnormalities of EFA metabolism may turn out to be one of the most common defects in human biochemistry and to be contributory causes in many human diseases," reported David F. Horrobin, Ph.D., and Mehar S. Manku in *Nutrition and Health,* a British publication. "Such abnormalities may occur for genetic reasons, as appears to be the case in allergy; for unknown reasons as in breast disease; as secondary consequences of other illnesses such as diabetes and alcoholism; and possibly because of aging and/or dietary indiscretions as in those at risk for cardiovascular disease."

They went on to say that patients with atopic eczema, premenstrual syndrome (PMS), or fibrocystic breast disease are apt to be deficient in one or more of the essential fatty acids.

"There is considerable clinical evidence that gamma-linolenic acid can correct some of the abnormalities in EFA patterns and can also lead to simultaneous clinical improvement, suggesting that the EFA abnormalities are playing a causative role," they continued.

## MAJOR ADVANCES

As Sinclair predicted 30 years ago, understanding of EFA metabolism seems likely to bring about major practical advances in clinical medicine.

Because of the complexity of the subject, this discussion will focus mainly on evening primrose oil, linseed/flaxseed oil and black currant seed oil. Depending on which part of the country you live in, linseed oil and flaxseed oil are often used synonymously as a nutritional supplement. This should not be confused with the boiled linseed oil sold in hardware stores as furniture polish.

As pointed out in *Natural Health, Natural Medicine* by Andrew Weil, M.D. (Houghton Mifflin, Boston, 1990), evening primrose oil, black currant oil and borage oil provide GLA, which is an effective anti-inflammatory agent with none of the side effects of anti-inflammatory drugs.

"It also promotes healthy growth of skin, hair and nails," Dr. Weil said. "I prescribe EFA frequently for skin conditions (including brittle nails and hair), arthritis, autoimmune disorders and premenstrual syndrome. Do not expect immediate results; it takes six to eight weeks to see changes after adding GLA to the diet. These three products vary in the amount of GLA they supply and in cost. I usually recommend black currant oil in doses of 500 milligrams twice a day as the most economical form."

In an unpublished study from England, 45 women with PMS began a treatment program consisting of 500-milligram capsules of black currant oil, four times daily, for 10 days prior to menstruation until the end of their period. Of those who completed the study, 36 percent reported a slight improvement in their symptoms, 20 percent said that some symptoms were gone; 29 percent reported most symptoms gone; and 4 percent said that all symptoms were gone. Eleven percent registered no improvement.

Researchers at the University of Rotterdam conducted a five-year study of one of the EFAs, linoleic acid, and showed that the diabetic complications of the heart, kidneys and eyes could be significantly reduced with regular doses, stated Robert C. Atkins, M.D. in *Dr. Atkins' Health Revolution* (Houghton Mifflin, Boston, 1988).

"Work in progress under the aegis of David F. Horrobin suggests that an even better effect can be achieved by GLA," Dr. Atkins said. "At any rate, fatty acids serving as precursors for beneficial prostaglandins hold great promise for helping ease the course of diabetes; their use must be considered in all diabetics."

## LOWERS "BAD" CHOLESTEROL

Research from several Japanese universities showed that evening primrose oil was effective in lowering low-density lipoprotein cholesterol, the so-called "bad" kind, in patients with hypercholesterolemia who did not have elevated triglyceride levels. Each volunteer received 3.6 grams of evening primrose oil daily. (*The Nutrition Report,* July 1989).

Believing that hyperactive children suffer from a deficiency of EFAs, researchers at the Hyperactive Children's Support Group in West Sussex, England, gave primrose oil to the children orally or rubbed it into the skin, since EFAs are rapidly absorbed into normal skin, according to Mark Bricklin in *The Practical Encyclopedia of Natural Healing* (Penguin, New York, 1990).

One of the participants, a 6-year-old boy, who was threatened with expulsion from school for his disruptive behavior, was given massages of evening primrose oil (1.5 grams) morning and night.

"The school was unaware of this," Bricklin said, "but after five days the teacher telephoned the mother and said that never in 30 years teaching had she seen such a dramatic change in a child's behavior. After three weeks the evening primrose oil was stopped, and one week later the school again complained. The oil was then reintroduced with good effect." Another boy, who was sensitive to wheat, could eat wheat again with no effects after EFA therapy, Bricklin said.

## HELP FOR MS PATIENTS

Research by Drs. Horrobin and Rudin has suggested that prostaglandins and their essential fatty acid precursors are involved with multiple sclerosis (MS) and that evening primrose oil has helped some patients. According to Abram Hoffer, M.D. Ph.D., in *Orthomolecular Medicine for Physicians* (Keats Publishing, New Canaan, CT, 1989), MS seems to be more prevalent in colder climates where more unsaturated fatty acids of the cold-weather type (fish oils and cold-weather plant oils such as flaxseed and canola) are required for optimal health. Yet our modern diet contains only 20 percent of the EFA it did 100 years ago.

## DULL, LIFELESS HAIR

Writing in *Dr. Wright's Guide to Healing with Nutrition* (Keats, New Canaan, CT, 1990), Jonathan V. Wright, M.D. said that anyone with dull, lifeless hair should reach for a bottle of flaxseed oil, rather than the latest miracle shampoo. Instead of dumping it on your head, you swallow about a tablespoon daily and see what happens in several weeks.

"Get a small bottle to minimize rancidity problems," Dr. Wright said. "Put 1,000 IUs of vitamin E into any opened bottle of oil to retard rancidity and keep refrigerated."

The best food source of essential fatty acids are those of food oils: fish, unroasted nuts, seeds and whole grains. Margarine and hydrogenated fats are detrimental and should be avoided.

To remain well, we need a variety of health-giving fats. Unfortunately, from the evidence, many of us are neglecting the important essential fatty acids.

# Natural Ways To Renew Dry Skin: Water, "Good" Fats Are Vital

*Vitamin A, B Complex, C and E Work To Moisturize; Oatmeal, Brewer's Yeast Provide Nourishing, Smoothing Facials*

People with dry skin do not produce enough sebum, the internal skin oil. This has an up side since excessive production of sebum is one of the basic causes of acne. People with dry skin are often spared the discomfort and misery of acne pimples. But later on, as the years advance, this plus turns into a minus, for the lack of lubrication from within the body can lead to a parched looking skin which wrinkles easily. But do not despair, there are solid nutritional and topical solutions to the problem.

## NUTRITIONAL SOLUTIONS

It is never too late to start on a constructive program of oiling and moisturizing your inner body and outer skin. Moisturize from within by drinking at least six to eight glasses of water each day, and feed your body and skin by taking one or another form of unsaturated fatty acid oils or gamma linolenic acid (GLA) found in evening primrose oil, which nourishes skin, hair and nails. Eat a wide variety of vitamin A, B complex, C and E-rich foods. If your skin is exceptionally dry, or if you are over forty years old, also add these same vitamins to your diet in the form of supplements, remembering that supplements are just what they say they are—and not substitutes for good food.

## TOPICAL SOLUTIONS

Many foods are moisturizing as well as nourishing and penetrating. For dry skin care this winter, try one of the following facials or masks:

### OATMEAL FACIAL

Super-fatted colloidal oatmeal makes a fine nourishing and bleaching facial base. To a tablespoon of oatmeal, add rosewater, nettle water, elder flower water or milk. Work material into a thick paste and gently pat on the neck and face. Allow the mask to dry for at least 15 minutes. Wash off with tepid water. The oatmeal creates a silken effect on the skin. Almond meal can be substituted for the oatmeal or added to the mask.

### BREWER'S YEAST FACIAL

A three-month "assault plan" would include drinking a tablespoon of this yeast in some strong juice such as apple, grape or cranberry each day, and applying the following mask once-a-week:

*few drops hot water*
*1 teaspoon honey*
*1 tablespoon brewer's yeast*
*1 teaspoon milk (or favorite skin oil)*
*1 teaspoon oil for face*

Add a few drops of hot water to honey to liquefy it. Blend in dried brewer's yeast. Add either milk or oil to soften. Stir into thick paste. Apply oil base to face. Pat paste on face. Allow to dry for 15 to 30 minutes. Remove with cotton ball or washcloth soaked in tepid water. Follow with a mild astringent such as cucumber, chamomile or witch hazel extract.

### VITAMIN A AND E FACIAL

Use this cream as a skin food after you have thoroughly cleansed your skin. Whenever possible use it an hour or two before you go to bed, then wipe off gently.

*1½ tablespoons beeswax*
*1 tablespoon white wax*
*1 tablespoon (liquid or solid) anhydrous lanolin*
*3 ounces sweet almond oil (avocado oil or safflower oil can also be used)*
*1 ounce distilled water*
*½ teaspoon borax*
*1 ounce rosewater (or use 2 ounces of rosewater and omit distilled water)*
*simple tincture of benzoin (not compound)*
*2 to 6 capsules (400 IU) vitamin E*
*2 to 6 capsules (25,000 IU) vitamin A*

In a double boiler, heat together the beeswax, the white wax and the lanolin. Slowly add almond, avocado or safflower oil. In a separate pan (glass or stainless steel) heat 1 ounce of distilled water; and the borax (this acts as a special emulsifier) until the borax dissolves completely. Slowly add the rose water so that it too is slightly warm. Now without allowing either pan to get cool, add the rose water and borax combination to the wax, lanolin and oil combination and beat with an electric beater for as long as it takes for the cream to cool to room temperature. Add the simple tincture of benzoin. Prick open your vitamin capsules, add to cream and beat until the vitamins are blended.

### HUMIDIFIERS

Unfortunately most apartments and houses are overheated in the wintertime. If you cannot regulate the heat yourself, purchase one or several small humidifiers for different rooms. These will release water back into the air. And remember, open the windows during wintertime. Don't live in an entirely sealed fortress without fresh air! This simple action can make you and your skin feel healthier.

DIAN DINCIN BUCHMAN, PH.D.

# Evening Primrose Oil Eases Symptoms of PMS, Cystic Mastitis; Strengthens Nails

*What You Should Know About This Natural Source of Gamma-Linolenic Acid (GLA)*

Evening primrose oil corrects several problems of special interest to women. If for no other reason, this may make evening primrose oil the best discovery of the century.

The pain of premenstrual tension is both physical and mental. Increased water retention swells tissues which results in abdominal pain and depression. Depression and irritability result from the brain swelling against the skull.

The gradual increase in fluid can produce pain and mood change beginning from two to 14 days before menstruation starts. Diuretics help reduce the build-up but care must be taken to assure an adequate intake of potassium and magnesium, which diuretics wash away.

## COMPLEX INTERACTIONS

Certain nutrients can bring relief naturally without the need for diuretics, and without the risk of mineral loss.

Vitamin B6 has been very effective in about 70% of women with premenstrual tension. Also vitamin E has helped many. And now we understand the interactions of vitamins B6, E, gamma-linolenic acid (GLA) and prostaglandins.

British studies have now found that evening primrose oil, the natural source of GLA, can relieve about 90 to 95% of women's premenstrual tension. They have found that evening primrose oil cures two-thirds of the women not helped by anything else, while another 20% were greatly improved.

The secret is not to wait until the discomfort begins but to take vitamin B6 and evening primrose oil daily. Many have found that 50 mg of vitamin

B6 and six 500 mg capsules of evening primrose oil daily are effective. The evening primrose oil capsules should be divided into two or three doses during the day. Extremely difficult cases may need a total of eight 500 mg capsules of evening primrose oil and up to 200 mg of vitamin B6. Vitamin E is generally helpful in the 100 to 600 mg range.

Evening primrose oil has also aided women with heavy and prolonged bleeding. Instead of a heavy blood loss for seven to ten days, their periods normalized to four or five days duration at normal blood loss. Relief should occur within two or three cycles.

The most common breast disease is cystic mastitis (also called benign breast disease) which affects about 20% of premenopausal women. Often cysts (lumps) are tender and painful especially prior to menstrual flow.

The cause of the cysts is thought to be an overproduction of the hormone prolactin, combined with a shortage of PGE. Evening primrose oil helps prevent cyst development and speedily removes existing lumps within a few months.

Vitamin E also helps this condition. A double-blind study led by Dr. Robert S. London at the Johns Hopkins University School of Medicine and Sinai Hospital in Baltimore found that 85% of women with advanced cases of the disease responded within eight weeks to 600 mg of vitamin E daily. In 40% of the women, there was a complete disappearance of the lumps.

The same regimen of evening primrose oil, vitamin B6 and vitamin E effective against premenstrual stress looks promising against cystic mastitis. Six to eight 500 mg capsules of evening primrose oil daily should, by itself, be effective for the vast majority of women. Stubborn cases may need the assist from the other vitamins.

Another surprising result of the research with evening primrose oil is that brittle fingernails harden and become normal within two to six weeks. This response is so consistent that it can be concluded that brittle nails are a newly recognized sign of essential fatty acid deficiency in humans. These findings have been published in the May 1981 issue of the *British Journal of Dermatology*. The benefit of this discovery is obvious to women, but also think about its potential use by doctors to diagnose essential fatty acid deficiency.

RICHARD A. PASSWATER, PH.D.

# FLAXSEED (LINSEED) OIL AND THE POWER OF OMEGA-3

*How to Make Nature's Cholesterol Fighters Work for You*

INGEBORG M. JOHNSTON, C.N. AND
JAMES R. JOHNSTON, PH.D.

A GOOD KIND OF FAT

With the increasing consumption of processed foods, our diets are becoming overloaded with omega-6 fatty acids at the expense of the beneficial omega-3 fatty acids, which are found primarily in flaxseed (linseed) and its oil, and in deep-water fish. Although they have been used therapeutically for over 5,000 years, scientists have fairly recently learned that flaxseed or flaxseed oil may lower blood cholesterol levels that are often associated with heart attacks and strokes, reduce the viscosity of blood, lower arterial blood pressure, prevent colon and breast cancer, improve moods, diminish allergies and produce a healthier skin. As detailed in this chapter, the increased consumption of omega-3 fatty acids from flaxseed/linseed products may provide protection against some major degenerative diseases.

## AN INTRODUCTION

Most people are interested in improving their personal health. This chapter is about a natural product that, in many cases, will help do just that. The product is a seed known as flaxseed or linseed.

Because of the confusion caused by the use of two different names, there has been an international effort to use the word "flaxseed" when referring to products from this plant that are produced for human consumption, and "linseed oil" when discussing products that have been denatured, made unfit for human consumption, and used commercially in paints, varnishes and the like. We will be discussing the seed and oil produced for human consumption, hence we will use the words flaxseed and flaxseed oil. Of course, old habits are hard to break, and some consumers still use the terms interchangeably.

What might flaxseed or flaxseed oil do for you? It may:

- Lower blood fat levels often associated with heart attacks and strokes
- Reduce harmful blood cholesterol levels with its soluble fibers
- Prevent colon and breast cancer through its rich source of lignins, a documented anticancer agent
- Improve moods, diminish allergies and produce a healthier skin

The denatured product, i.e., linseed oil, can be used as a paint-reducer, a wood preservative, an oil stain and a concrete sealer. Linseed oil is also found in printing inks, putty, caulking materials, gum erasers, brake linings and hardboard, and is the main ingredient in linoleum, a term taken from the word linseed.

This chapter is about flaxseed and flaxseed oil, sometimes called "nutritional gold," which have a very important component: omega-3 fatty acid or linolenic acid.

Flaxseed has existed for 5,000 years, but it has been only recently that its benefits have been scientifically documented and shown to be effective in improving general health.

Carbohydrates, fats and proteins are the three energy nutrients. Carbohydrates have received the most attention in the short history of what might be called the Era of Nutritional Sciences, which began in the early 1900s. Next on the research list for studies were the proteins and their components, the amino acids. Only relatively recently have lipids, commonly called fats, taken the study and research spotlight . . . and with extraordinary results.

This chapter will:

- Review the reasons for an interest in fats
- Explain some of what has been learned about fats
- Define and develop the dietary concepts of polyunsaturated fatty acids
- Discuss some of the contributions and dramatic impact that flaxseed and its by-products—flaxseed oil and flaxseed meal—are making

In addition, this chapter will support the following:

1. The hypothesis that Donald O. Rudin, M.D., an American medical researcher, has established regarding the existence of an inverse relationship between the increased consumption of processed foods and the decreased consumption of omega-3 oils, an important component of flaxseed.
2. The argument that Dr. Johanna Budwig, a German Nobel Prize nominee, has developed, that many contemporary diseases result from fatty degeneration and essential fatty acid deficiencies.

If these two recognized experts are correct in their positions, then the logical conclusion might be that too much of the "wrong" kinds of fats and oils and too little of the "right" essential kinds of fats and oils, such as flaxseed, are being consumed today.

As the saying goes, there is nothing so powerful as an idea whose time has come. Perhaps for the reasons reviewed in this chapter the time for flaxseed has indeed arrived.

## THE CHOLESTEROL AGE

We live in what might be called the Cholesterol Age. Almost everyone knows something about the fat known as cholesterol. Some of this information is correct and some of it is not. It would seem that hardly a day goes by that we don't read articles or watch news features about what cholesterol substances do in the body, about what one is supposed to do if these cholesterol levels are too high and about the impact of cholesterol from the foods we eat. Many of these reports fail to mention that the body *normally produces* varying amounts of this fat each day.

The preponderance of information that we see and read generally supports the concept that dietary cholesterol plays a role in the development of coronary heart disease (CHD). CHD is one of the major health problems in the United States and includes atherosclerosis, hypertension, altered blood platelet functions and ischemia (deficiency of blood to the heart muscle).

New information on the role of essential fatty acids, that is, fatty acids that our bodies cannot produce, is causing a renewed interest in just how much fat we eat and in the composition of that fat. In the past, the food and pharmaceutical industries have sold us on the importance of replacing lard, a fat that is solid at room temperature and is very low in essential fatty acids, with such oils as sunflower, safflower or corn, fats that are liquid at room temperature and contain essential fatty acids which our body cannot produce.

We have learned from researchers that there are two kinds of essential fatty acids and that, while we have been getting more than our share of the omega-6 fatty acids found in such warm-weather plant seeds as sunflower, safflower and corn oils, we have not been getting enough omega-3 fatty acids, found in cold-water fatty fish and in certain cold-weather plant seeds like flaxseed.

## HEALTH STATUS U.S.A.

In 1977, the Secretary of Health, Education and Welfare, Joseph Califano, stated that something had to be done about health-care costs in America, which were $229 billion annually or more than $1,000 per person.[1] Something has been done, but not what Mr. Califano had in mind. By 1989, the health-care figures had ballooned to almost $1.5 billion a day, twice the 1977 figure. Since then the amount of dollars spent on medical care has increased by exorbitant amounts.

Moreover, the number of people involved in providing health care in the United States, over five million, makes it one of the largest industries in the country, along with manufacturing, the wholesale/retail trade and travel.

Based on these expenditures, citizens of the United States should be the healthiest people in the world. No other country spends such enormous amounts, actual or per capita, on the health of its citizens. Are we getting our money's worth? Few people would say yes. And statistics on the rank of the United States healthwise among countries of the world support this feeling.

When the state of health care in America is discussed today, there is increasingly more recognition that improvements in health may result not from improving the medical care delivery system that has been used the past 60 years, but from efforts to promote health through changes in personal life-style and the environment and to focus on preventative health care rather than treatment-based medical care.

M. A. Caliendo states that nutrition is perhaps the most easily modified environmental factor that can directly contribute to improved health.[2] If national nutrition habits can be modified fairly easily, then a review of studies on the economic effects of good versus poor nutrition will make clear that this is an area that deserves more consideration.

## THE COST OF POOR NUTRITION

Nutrition is a relatively new science. The first broad scientific studies of nutrition and malnutrition in the United States took place in 1970. The Ten-State Survey and the Health and Nutrition Examination Survey (HANES) showed the prevalence of malnutrition and pointed out that many U.S. citizens were approaching that condition.[3]

Malnutrition in Western cultures is characterized by "overnutrition," which is basically an excess of food intake. Many health and medical experts believe that excess food intake leads to obesity and other diseases specific to Western civilized countries.

The results of the surveys and comments of these experts may be summarized this way:

> There is an overconsumption of fat in general and specifically saturated fat, as well as cholesterol, sugar, salt and alcohol; all of these have been associated with major diseases that have caused death and disability in the United States.[4,5]

If this evaluation is accurate, then simple changes in life-style and consumption habits could significantly reduce the susceptibility to and/or the progression of potentially fatal disorders like coronary heart disease, high blood pressure, diabetes mellitus, dental caries, liver disease and obesity.[6] If the logical conclusion from surveys and experts is that the cost of poor nutrition is high, what could be the savings of good nutrition?

## THE ECONOMIC BENEFIT OF GOOD NUTRITION

B. Popkin developed a model to determine the economic costs of malnutrition, in which the economic benefits from improved nutrition were revealed in five major areas:[7]

| | |
|---|---|
| Education | —\$6.4–19.2 billion |
| Physical performance | —\$6.4–25.8 billion |
| Morbidity | —\$201–502 billion |

| | |
|---|---|
| Mortality | —$68–157 billion |
| Intergeneration effects | —$1.3–4.5 billion |

The above figures should be higher because some costs that were difficult to evaluate were excluded, but the magnitude of the problem and the value of improving nutrition is apparent.

The USDA conducted a study in 1971 that estimated that dramatic savings from major health problems would take place if diets were improved.[8] Examples included reduction of heart and vascular problems by 25 percent; reduction of the number of people with arthritis by 50 percent; and reduction of the number of deaths and acute conditions from cancer by 20 percent.

Another study based on data from the U.S. Department of Agriculture estimated that improved nutritional status of North Americans might reduce the national health bill by one-third.[9] The study suggested that, based on conservative scientific opinion, over $40 billion a year could be saved in such areas as dental caries, diabetes, cardiovascular disease, alcoholism and digestive diseases.

The high costs of poor nutrition on one side, and the economic benefits of good nutrition on the other, would seem to encourage national concern for the concept that better nutrition is a viable, low-tech, affordable way to attain the goal of improving the health status of the general public.

## CHANGES IN FOOD CONSUMPTION OVER A CENTURY

Since the beginning of the century, dramatic changes in food consumption in the United States have taken place. While you may be aware that fruits, grains and vegetables, which were once an important part of the dinner table, have been replaced by fat and refined sugar, you may not be aware of the extent to which that has happened. Some nutrition reviews state that approximately 60 percent of the calories of the average American's diet today comes from fats and refined sugars.[10]

Since the concern here is with fat, let's examine some facts about fat. In 1909, the average person in the United States consumed about 125 grams of fat per day. Today the consumption is closer to 175 grams, a daily increase of 40 percent and an annual increase of approximately 50 pounds. Rudin states that fat consumption rose from about 33 percent of total calories daily to almost 50 percent, and is still increasing.[11] Of the total increase in the consumption of fats and oils, shortening, margarine, refined salad oil and cooking oils account for 50 percent.

Further, a shift in the kinds of fat consumed is also evident. It has been shown that about 42 percent of total dietary calories come from fat (16 percent saturated fat, 7 percent polyunsaturated fat and 19 percent from monounsaturated fat).

Historical studies have shown that there has been a significant increase in the consumption of polyunsaturated fats as well. In 1909, the ratio of polyunsaturated fat to saturated fat (P/S) was P21/S100 or 0.21. In the 1980s, the ratio has changed to P43/S100 or 0.43. This increase is easy to understand when one realizes that 80 percent of the total fat intake in our diets today is derived from vegetable oils, which are mostly polyunsaturated.[12]

If the vegetable oils are mostly unsaturated and if there is a relationship between heart attacks and saturated fat consumption, why do we not have fewer heart attacks than when we were consuming more saturated fats? The answer is not a simple one because on one hand we are still consuming too much *overall* fat and on the other there seems to be a trend toward fewer heart attacks.

The American Heart Association recommends a P/S ratio of approximately one-to-one.[13] While we are getting closer to this ratio, this same group suggests that the *total* percent of all calories from fat should be reduced to 20 percent of the total calories (10 percent saturated fat and 10 percent unsaturated fat), which we are getting farther and farther away from.

The publication entitled "Straight Talk About Fat and Your Health" suggests that we should consider a "Dietary Fat Equation."[14]

The basis of the equation is emphasis on fresh, natural and unrefined foods, thus effectively lowering the intake of fat quantity while elevating the intake of fat quality. Examples include:

| DECREASE (or eliminate) the bad fats | INCREASE the good fats |
|---|---|
| margarine | whole grains |
| shortening | seeds |
| butter | beans |
| prepared meats | fresh vegetables |
| dairy products | low-fat dairy products |
| salad dressings | seafood/sea vegetables |
| chips (corn, potato) | lean meat (skinless chicken) |
| fried foods | |
| pastry | |

We have reviewed the health status of the United States and considered the argument for the value of changing nutrition and life-style habits. In doing this, we have used terminology with which you may not be familiar. In order to understand the important role that flaxseed can play, we need to define some of the terms.

## DEFINITIONS—WORDS, CONCEPTS AND TERMS

**Fat.** Fat is a common word used interchangeably with the scientific term "lipid." Members of the lipid family include triglycerides (about 95 percent of fats in the body are triglycerides), phospholipids (an example is lecithin) and sterols (an example is cholesterol). Fats are used in the body as:

- Carriers of essential nutrients, such as essential fatty acids and fat-soluble vitamins
- Concentrated form of energy when stored as body fat
- Insulation against cold or protection against injury

- A carbohydrate-sparing nutrient which can also be converted to protein
- Satiety enhancer in food (makes us feel full)
- Taste improver in foods (don't we know it!)

Fat is a chemical combination of carbon, hydrogen and oxygen and, when compared to carbohydrate and protein, the other energy sources in the body, it provides twice as many calories per molecule. It is hydrophobic or not compatible with water, a fact that is important when we wonder how fats can be transported in the blood, which is mostly water.

**Fatty Acids (FAs).** Fatty acids are chemical compositions composed of a chain of carbons attached to each other with a carboxyl or acid group on one end. Think of a snake whose body is the carbon chain, which does not like water (hydrophobic), and whose head is the acid group, which likes water (hydrophilic). The snake has both "fat"—the carbon chain body, and acid—the head; hence the term "fatty acid."

FA chains can be short, medium or long, depending on how many carbon atoms are linked to each other in the snake's body. A FA with over 12 carbons in the chain is considered a long-chain FA.

**Saturated Fatty Acids (SFAs).** Certain FAs can be saturated with hydrogen. When the carbon elements in the chain cannot hold any more hydrogen, the molecule is considered saturated, hence the term, saturated fatty acids. Carbons in the carbon chains of SFAs are attached to each other by means of a single bond. Lard and shortening are examples of saturated fat.

**Unsaturated Fatty Acids (UFAs).** Some FAs are not saturated with hydrogen. Generally, any fatty acid that has carbon chains which could hold more hydrogen is called an unsaturated fatty acid. Some carbons in the carbon chains of UFAs are attached to each other by what are called "double bonds," as opposed to one bond, as in the SFA. Under certain conditions double bonds can be separated to take on extra hydrogen. Compounds with double bonds are much more active than compounds with single bonds, which are fairly inert.

A fatty acid chain with one double bond is called a monounsaturated fat (example: oleic acid in olive oil). If the fatty chain has more than one double bond, it is called a polyunsaturated fat or PUFA. Most unsaturated fatty acids are PUFAs.

Again, UFAs are more unstable, more chemically reactive and tend to be more physiologically beneficial than SFAs. UFAs are the subject of most concern in this chapter.

The length of the fatty acid chain—short, medium or long—and the saturated or unsaturated nature of the fatty acid are two important concepts. They determine how easily the FA can be absorbed by the body (the shorter chain fatty acids are absorbed more easily). The oils, usually liquid at room temperature and unsaturated, are absorbed better than the fats, which are generally solid at room temperature.

**Essential Fatty Acids (EFAs).** The term EFA suggests that there are certain fatty acids essential to the body and that is correct. Like other essential nutrients not produced in the body, EFAs must be ingested.

Linoleic acid (LA) is an essential fatty acid, because the body cannot produce its own supply. LA is an 18 carbon-chain fatty acid with two double bonds starting from the sixth carbon in the chain. In technical shorthand, LA would be 18:2w6. Because the first double bond starts at the sixth carbon in the chain, LA belongs to the omega-6 family.

Another EFA that has been considered essential is alpha linolenic acid (LNA or ALENA). Because the body does make some LNA from LA, some experts do not consider it to be an essential fatty acid. Whether it is essential or not, it is most important. LNA is an 18 carbon chain with three double bonds starting from the third carbon in the chain. In technical shorthand LNA would be 18:3w3.

Functions of EFAs include:

- Regulation of cholesterol metabolism
- Maintainence and regulation of the functions and integrity of all cell membranes which are composed primarily of fat
- Serving as precursors to very active, hormone-like substances such as prostaglandins, which scientists have found over the past 30

years regulate nearly every body function; and thromboxanes and prostacyclins, which are important to the health of the arteries.

**Cholesterol and Total Cholesterol.** As we have learned, cholesterol is a fat from the sterol family and it is a normal constituent of blood and tissue. Cholesterol is present in all animal fat and oil, bile, brain tissue, blood and egg yolk. It is a derived lipid, which means that it is a compound composed of a fat and an active acetate called CoA or Co-enzyme A. Cholesterol can be made from carbohydrates, fats or proteins.

Total cholesterol is made up of a number of components. Unless otherwise stated, the word cholesterol usually means total cholesterol, that is, all of the cholesterol components taken together. There are two important components of total cholesterol.

**Cholesterol—HDL (High-Density Lipoproteins).** HDLs (called good cholesterol) carry unused cholesterol out of the arteries. You could think of them as the garbage collectors. They are less dense because they have less lipids and more protein than the LDLs.

**Cholesterol—LDL (Low-Density Lipoproteins).** LDLs deliver cholesterol from the liver into the bloodstream. As you might expect, because of the job they do, they are composed of more lipids and less protein than the HDLs.

The functions of LDLS include:

- Facilitating the absorption of fatty acids
- Transporting fatty acids in the bloodstream
- Being a basic ingredient in the formation of bile salts, vitamin D, and certain hormones (adrenal, steroid and sex)

**Lipids.** "Lipids" is the scientific term for fats. They are usually defined in terms of solubility. If a substance is not soluble in water but is soluble in fatty substances and organic (composed partially of carbon atoms) solvents, it is considered a lipid.

Lipids are divided into three categories: simple, compound and derived.

**Simple Lipids.** Simple lipids are called true or neutral fats and include fatty acids and the mono-, di- and triglycerides. The mono- and diglycerides are not common in foods but are significant commercially because they make hydrogenated products like shortening more plastic or pliable.

Triglycerides (TGs) are composed of one glycerol and three fatty acid molecules hooked together. TGs serve as the major form of storage of fatty acids and are almost the exclusive constituent of adipose tissue.

**Compound Lipids.** Compound lipids are different from simple lipids in that they contain a nonlipid portion. Compound lipids are usually special molecules that are used to accomplish specific functions.

Compound lipids include a two-part molecule, e.g.:

- A fatty acid and a phosphorus-containing group, as in lecithin, which helps to regulate cell permeability
- A fatty acid and a carbohydrate group, as in glycolipids, which function in the nerve tissues
- A fatty acid and a protein group, as in lipoproteins which are compounds that have a lipid in the center and a protein coating. Since protein reacts well to water, the molecule can be transported easily in the bloodstream, which would not be the case if the lipid were not protein-coated.

**Derived Lipids.** Derived lipids include fatty acids and other compounds that are actually or potentially related to active acetate or CoA, Co-Enzyme A, as stated earlier. Steroids are classified as derived lipids and the best known steroid is cholesterol.

**Cisoid or Cis Fats.** The natural configuration for a fatty acid is the cis form. In this form, hydrogen atoms, which tend to repel each other, are on the same side of a carbon double bond, which causes the carbon chain to bend away from the hydrogen side.

**Transoid or Trans Fats.** The trans fats configuration is an unnatural form brought about by high temperatures or other factors. The hydrogen atoms are on opposite sides of the carbon chain and since there is not the repelling force as in the cis fats, the molecule tends to remain straight. None of the trans-forms of a molecule are biologically equivalent to the parent molecule.

## THE IMPORTANCE OF THE OMEGA-3 FATTY ACID FAMILY

Paul Stitt, a biochemist and international authority on flax, reported to a conference of flax producers in 1988 that, with all of the research now being done on fatty acids, there are about 200 studies published per month on the subject, and that there are more than 350,000 catalogued studies on lipids and fats.[15]

Manufacturers in and suppliers to the natural foods industry have collected thousands of studies that go back to the 1950s on the fatty acids in marine oils alone.

The Flax Institutes of Canada and the United States are valuable sources of research and information, as are the producers and suppliers of flaxseed oil in both countries. These individuals and groups are mentioned to show the present interest in learning more about fats, and to indicate that there are hundreds of recent studies available, if one wishes to become better informed in this area.

Flaxseed is relevant to fat studies because two of its components, LA and LNA, are essential fatty acids. Flaxseed also has one of the highest amounts of LNA of any natural product.[16]

Both LA and LNA are included in the 50 or so essential nutrients that the body cannot produce. Both react easily to other substances in the body. Each is employed by the body in different ways to maintain health.

The average diet does not include foods that are high in omega-3 components. Omega-3 fatty acids are primarily found in seeds and plants from cold climates, green leafy vegetables and in oils extracted from cold-water fish like mackerel, salmon, tuna or cod.

With the advent of mass food merchandising and the subsequent processing of foods, most of what the average person eats is processed or otherwise changed from its original form. To add to this problem, there has been a concerted effort to remove all the omega-3 components from our foods to keep them from spoiling and to extend shelf life. Foods that contain omega-3 oils spoil easily, because the unsaturated fatty acids attract oxygen and become oxidized or turn rancid. Ironically, this feature of attracting oxygen easily is the reason that unsaturated fatty acids are so important to our health, because they help carry oxygen in the body.

While food processing removes as much of the omega-3 components as possible, whatever is left is probably totally destroyed through hydrogenation. Hydrogenation is a hydrogen-adding process that changes the unsaturated, easily spoiled liquid oils into more saturated or solid products with longer shelf lives. A final product example is margarine.

Prehistoric human diets and traditional agricultural diets contained considerably more omega-3 oils than the contemporary diet of people in industrialized nations.[17] As previously mentioned, Rudin documented the declining intake of the omega-3 fatty acids during the twentieth century. He theorized that this decline has contributed to the origin and development of diseases whose incidence has been increasing during this century. Rudin argues that there is a relationship between modern major illnesses and unrecognized nutritional diseases, which he believes are caused, at least in part, by an undersupply of the omega-3 oils.

In 1980, Sinclair reported evidence that omega-3 EFA deficiencies and excess saturated fat consumption were related to cardiovascular disease,[18] a view now espoused by many heart and cancer panels.[19]

In 1953, Budwig reported that she could change the yellow-green protein substance in the blood to healthy red blood pigment or hemoglobin by giving cancer patients four ounces of nonfat cottage cheese and three tablespoons of fresh flax oil per day for three months. She also reported that proper lipoproteins and phosphatides, previously lacking, reappeared following treatment with the dietary supplement.

This would suggest that the blood of these cancer patients was deficient in essential fatty acids, phosphatides and albumin (a blood protein). The deficiency stopped when EFAs were carried directly into the bloodstream, bypassing the liver, with the help of the sulfur-rich amino acids from the protein in the cottage cheese.[20]

The Gerson Institute has experimented with oils in the diets of their patients for many years and now uses flax oil daily for their cancer patients.[21]

Reviewing what EFAs do in the body and recognizing some of the symptoms, problems and deficiencies of modern degenerative diseases, lend support to the positions taken by Budwig, Rudin, Sinclair and others.

## BENEFITS OF THE OMEGA-3 AND OMEGA-6 FATTY ACIDS

By regulating cholesterol metabolism, including transportation, conversion to other substances, storage and excretion, omega-3 and omega-6 fatty acids help HDL cholesterol molecules to travel smoothly through the bloodstream and assist in the conversion into bile salts. This is the only way for the body to get rid of cholesterol. Without this process working properly, susceptibility to degenerative heart and artery conditions is dramatically increased.

Omega-3 and -6 help stabilize and strengthen all cell membranes, making them more fluid and flexible. Enhanced fluidity and flexibility of cell membranes facilitates effective exchange of materials between the inner and outer cell membrane layers. Efficient transport of materials is needed for new tissue construction and tissue repair.

Since experts say that unhealthy or leaky cells are the basis of many problems ranging from allergies to cancer to the level of activity of the immune system, anything that will strengthen the cell walls is important. The omega-3 and omega-6 fatty acid families do just that.

Omega-3 and -6 are constituents of the raw materials or precursors to prostaglandins, which are very active biological substances that regulate nearly every body function including:

- The inflammatory process
- The healing and repair process
- The immune system
- The neural circuits in the brain

- The cardiovascular system (including cholesterol levels and actions in the bloodstream)
- The digestive and reproductive systems
- The body thermostat and calorie-loss mechanism.[22]

By controlling the relationships between the organ-level hormones and the enzymes in the various cells, they can reduce the chances for hormone-irregularity diseases.

By providing the fluidity needed for proper reception and transmission of impulses between the brain cells, they can control brain functions. Of the many complex fatty acids in the human brain, the most abundant polyunsaturated fatty acid is DHA (docosahexaenoic acid), an omega-3 family member with a 22 carbon chain. It is a derivative of omega-3 LNA.

Lack of EFA can cause a reduction in number and size of brain cells as well as a lack of communication between the brain cells and can involve problems in learning, growing and thinking.

Given the extensive overall regulatory role of the omega-6 and omega-3 families, it can be seen how their low levels could disrupt body functions and produce problems that result in or are related to today's modern degenerative conditions.

Rudin contends that while the levels of omega-6 fatty acids (mostly warm-weather vegetable oils) have increased in our diets, the levels of omega-3 fatty acids have been reduced some 80 percent in the past hundred years. If this is the case, then it should follow that at least part of the reason for our increase in degenerative diseases is our low consumption of omega-3 fatty oils.

## STUDIES SUPPORT THE VALUE OF OMEGA-3 FATTY ACIDS

The March 3, 1988 issue of the *New England Journal of Medicine* included the article, "Medical Progress—Cardiovascular Effect on n-3 (Omega-3) Fatty Acids" by Leaf and Weber. It is an excellent summary of recent studies on omega-3 oils focusing primarily on fish oils. Simopolous, who organized the NATO Advanced Research Workshop on "Dietary Omega 3 and 6 Fatty Acids" in Italy in 1988, wrote a comprehensive article that appeared in the March/April and May/June 1988 issues of *Nutrition Today.*

A good place to begin is with Dr. J. Dyerberg, who is perhaps the world's leading authority on omega-3 fatty acids in marine oils. His group conducted studies in the late 1970s on the diet of the Greenland Eskimos which showed that Eskimos had low levels of low-density lipoproteins (LDL, the bad cholesterol carriers) and high levels of high-density lipoproteins (HDL, the good cholesterol carriers) despite eating a high fat diet of fatty fish and seals.[23]

Dyerberg's study led to diet and blood lipid comparison studies with Eskimos and people from Denmark, eating what we would call more normal diets. (The Danes came out second with higher LDLs, higher total cholesterol and significantly lower HDLs.) Further studies showed the beneficial effects of fish and fish-oil supplements on plasma lipid levels. It was generally concluded that DHA (docosahexaenoic acid, 22 carbon chain) and EPA (eicosapentaenoic acid, 20 carbon chain), both from the omega-3 fatty acid family, were responsible for these results.

Dyerberg's observations on the effects of omega-3 fatty acids on lipids included:

- Lowering levels of total cholesterol and low-density cholesterol
- Changing eicosanoids (special mission fatty acids) in a beneficial manner
- Reducing viscosity of whole blood
- Possibly lowering arterial blood pressure.

Research studies using flaxseed oil, with its high levels of omega-3 fatty acids (LNA), yielded some of the same results. This makes sense when we realize that the body can change LNA, an 18 carbon chain fatty acid, into EPA, a 20 carbon chain, and into DHA, a 22 carbon chain, all in the omega-3 family, through a step or pathway process.

The following list presents examples of research published in scientific literature that would seem to support the benefits of essential fatty acids in flaxseed:

1. In Great Britain, Sinclair in 1984 conducted specific research and concluded that, "A deficiency of essential fatty acids in experimental animals causes lesions, mainly attributable to faulty cellular membranes, sudden failure of growth, lesions of skin and kidney and connective tissue, erythrocyte fragility and impaired fertility."[24]

   Sinclair determined that a relative deficiency of the essential fatty acids was common in Western diets and that this deficiency played an important part in the causes of arteriosclerosis, coronary thrombosis, multiple sclerosis, diabetes mellitus, hypertension and certain forms of malignant diseases.
2. Again in Great Britain, Saynor, in a study of 92 people who had heart disease, found that sufficient omega-3 fatty acids in the diet rapidly reduced serum triglyceride levels and increased high-density lipoprotein (HDL—the good cholesterol).[25]
3. In Canada, Horrobin in 1980 found that alcohol does its damage to the fetus and to the liver by interfering with normal essential fatty acid metabolism.[26]
4. In the United States, Rudin found that omega-3 fatty acid deficiency is the basic cause of major mental illness because that fatty acid provides the substrate upon which niacin and other B vitamins act to form the prostaglandin-3 series tissue hormones (special mission fatty acids) which regulate neurocircuits through the whole body.[27]
5. Again in the United States, Dr. Patricia Johnston found that a diet containing 10 percent linseed oil could drastically change the prostaglandin content of serum and the fatty acid content of human breast milk by a factor of ten, within five days.[28]
6. In Poland, a research project concluded with the summary, "Fatty acids isolated from linseed oil were found to exhibit a

strong cytotoxic (cell destroying) *in vitro* (outside the body) activity, against (certain) cancer cells with minimal cytotoxic effect on normal cells (leukocytes) of rabbits. The fatty acids from linseed oil (1,000 g/ml after a three-hour incubation) gave 100-percent dead carcinoma cells.[29]

7. In 1981, a research project from Australia used low concentrations of linseed oil and linolenic acid to successfully combat strep infection in hospitals in Victoria.[30]
8. In Germany, "A diet of linseed oil (30 ml daily) for four weeks raised the content of LNA by 200 percent, the level of EPA by 150 percent and the level of DHA by 70 percent. The human body seems capable of transforming linolenic acid into EPA. This change coincided with a significantly reduced production of platelet thromboxanes (clotting agents)."[31]
9. In 1982, Dr. J. R. Vane shared the Nobel Prize for Medicine for his work in showing how the metabolism of omega-3 fatty acids helped to prevent heart problems.
10. In 1988, Dr. Stephen Cunnane, a University of Toronto professor, presented results at a meeting of the Canadian Flax Council that indicated that flax (linseed) contains insoluble fiber which reduces insulin secretion, giving it a very positive potential for use in a dietary intervention plan for diabetes. Fiber has been shown to have a strongly beneficial effect on glucose-tolerance curves.[32]
11. A study in the United States, by Chowdhury and Chandra, resulted in the observations that "alterations in lipid metabolism or intake affect the immune system in addition to other bodily tissues. In animals, deficiency of essential fatty acids depresses antibody response to T cells (protector cells), and dependent and independent antigens (foreign substances that stimulate an immune response)."[33] This study suggests a positive relationship between fatty acids and areas of immune system efficacy.
12. For the aspirin-a-day people, Von Schacky completed a study in 1988 that concludes with the comment that ". . . omega-3 fatty

acids induce favorable alterations in blood lipids, platelet responsiveness, blood pressure and response to pressor hormones (those that raise blood pressure and constrict arteries), and eicosanoid (special mission fatty acids) formations. These omega-3 fatty acids may be more effective in primary and secondary prophylaxis than aspirin."[34]

13. *Nutritional Influences on Illness, A Sourcebook of Clinical Research,* by Melvyn R. Werbach, M.D. (Keats Publishing, New Canaan, Conn. 1988), cites research involving some 26 diseases, ranging from acne vulgaris to tardive dyskinesia, which were helped in some way by the omega-3 fatty acids.

## FLAXSEED OIL AND FLAXSEED MEAL—THE OTHER COMPONENTS

An argument has developed that sets forth the importance of increasing the amounts of omega-3 oils in our diets. Flaxseed, with approximately 60 percent LNA, is probably the best source of omega-3 oils. What else does flaxseed have to offer?

Looking at the other components of flaxseed oil, we find that:

- 16 percent is LA, the double-unsaturated, omega-6 fatty acid
- 18 percent is oleic acid, the monounsaturated, omega-9 fatty acid
- Other nutrients present include vitamin E and beta-carotene, a precursor to vitamin A

Looking at the other components of flaxseed meal, and particularly of ground fortified flax for human consumption, we find:

- High levels of calcium, magnesium, manganese and potassium
- High levels of soluble fiber. Soluble fiber is known to reduce blood cholesterol. Typical of investigations in this area is one by S. Cunnane, who used flaxseed in a diet study that produced a 27 percent reduction in blood cholesterol.[35] Studies have also shown the relation between soluble fiber and lowering the incidence of colon and breast cancer.

- Lignins, documented anti-cancer agents[36]
- Protein, which suggests that flax could be substituted for other forms of protein that contain less healthy forms of fat, such as pork and beef.

## FLAXSEED MEAL FED TO ANIMALS

Why should we be interested in the results of feeding animals flaxseed? The fat found in most of the animal meats consumed by the average American is saturated fat. Relationships between the consumption of saturated fat and degenerative diseases like heart problems have been well established. It might be speculated that feeding flaxseed, which we have learned contains the good fats—omega-3, omega-6 and omega-9—to chickens, cows and pigs, could change the kinds of fat found in these animals from mostly saturated to mostly unsaturated.[37] Thus when people eat the meat from these animals, they might get less saturated fat and more unsaturated fat into their systems. More research would seem to be in order in this area.

There are other changes in the animals that can be attributed to the use of flaxseed in the diet. Stitt refers to a study in which one group of chickens was fed flaxmeal and another group regular chicken feed. The flaxmeal group grew twice as fast with stronger bones (perhaps an implication for use with osteoporosis) than those fed regular chicken feed.[38]

The Flax Council of Canada suggests that a change in the composition of fat from bad fats to good fats in the products of dairy cattle might be effected by feeding them more crushed flaxseed because of the omega-3 fatty acids in the flaxmeal. The argument for changes in the fat in the milk from saturated to unsaturated would be the same as outlined previously.

A unique factor about flaxseed is its ability to act in a gentle, regulating way upon the digestive system. Flaxseed absorbs up to eight times its own weight in water and, because of its high mucilage content, improves digestion in livestock. It has also been reported that flaxseed is responsible for removing toxic metabolites produced during digestion and reducing the occurrence of bloat. Perhaps this is the reason that farmers fed their cattle cooked flax cake before the use of antibiotics.

## GROWING FLAXSEED

Cultivated flax belongs to the species *Linum usitatissimum.* There are two main varieties, one which is grown for oil and one which is grown for fiber production.

Flax seeds are flat, oval and pointed at one end. A thousand seeds weigh from 4.5 to 7.0 grams. Seeds range in color from light to dark reddish brown or yellow. The seed is covered with a mucilaginous coating that imparts a high gloss and causes the seed to become sticky when wet.

In North America, the market for yellow-seeded or golden flax is limited to organic health food products. Most of the yellow-seeded flax grown in Canada is exported to the European Economic Community and used primarily as a topping in the food industry. Flax oil is common in Europe and was common in the United States until the beginning of World War II.

Flax is an annual plant grown mostly in the colder regions of the world. Canada is the world leader in high-quality flax production. The high quality results from the high oil content, the high iodine value, which measures the relative drying or oxidizing quality, important when it is used in paints and varnishes, and the fact that Canadian-grown flax is the best source of LNA, grown out-of-doors, in the world.

Part of the reason for the high quality of the flax grown in Canada is the cool, long days common to the northern latitudes, which increase the levels of fatty acids and oils in the seeds. Eighty-five percent of the world's flaxseed production is concentrated in Canada, the United States, Argentina, India and the former Soviet Union.

## PROCESSING

### FLAXSEED OIL

The advantages of flaxseed oil are found only if the oil remains fresh; it is a perishable product and must be protected not only during the processing but also during the handling and storing. Enemies of fresh flaxseed oil are oxygen (exclusion prevents oxidation or rancidity), light (exclusion prevents free-radical formation), and heat (exclusion prevents trans-fatty acid formation).

In order for flaxseed oil to be effective, it must be cold-pressed below 40°C., unrefined, unfiltered and nondeodorized. Because of these needs, mass processing methods are usually not acceptable.

### FLAXSEED (LINSEED) MEAL

The flaxseed is crushed for feed to livestock. The linseed meal or oil cake is composed of 40 percent protein, of which 85 percent is digestible. Since the crushed flaxseed is deficient in the amino acid lysine, it is limited as a sole source of protein and, therefore, must be mixed with grains or other feed.

### FORTIFIED FLAXSEED MEAL

Some manufacturers have developed a process of crushing the flaxseed without losing the nutrients. Next, the crushed flaxseed is fortified with zinc, iron, niacin (B3), B6 and B12. This meal thus provides a food for humans that has all of the advantages of flaxseed discussed in this booklet and none of the disadvantages, like quick rancidity and free radical or trans-fatty acid formation when light, heat and air are not excluded.

## HANDLING AND STORING

**Flaxseed** is fairly durable and can be handled like most grains. Strains have been developed to resist rust and wilt. There is a problem with the mucilaginous coating that causes the seed to become sticky when it gets wet or swells and bursts during periods of prolonged rainfall or high humidity. While this is a problem when the flaxseed is being stored, it is a boon to people who are trying to regulate their bowel function. This swelling in the intestinal tract provides easy bulk which stimulates bowel functioning.

**Flaxseed oil** must be handled carefully. To insure flaxseed oil freshness, heat, light and air (oxygen) must be eliminated during the processing and storage phases.

## COFACTORS FOR BETTER METABOLISM

Flax contains an anti-B6 factor that Dr. Klosterman from North Dakota State University has identified.[37] Very small amounts of B6 should be taken to overcome this factor. In addition, there are insufficient amounts of zinc, iron, niacin (B3), B6 and B12. In order for the omega-3 oils to be maximally utilized, these nutrients are added to fortified flaxmeal.

## CAUTIONS

The following are some points to be kept in mind when using flax.

- Omega-3 oils greatly increase the effectiveness of the B-complex vitamins, so megadoses of these vitamins should be avoided.
- Do not use flaxseed oil in deep frying. Frying destroys the oil and can produce toxic substances. While flax oil can be used in dough for baking, it cannot be used for basting, grilling or lining pans. It's good for salads and flaxseed bread, which is common in Europe.

- Flaxseed contains glycoside linamarin, which can release hydrocyanic acid (cyanide) in the acidic gastric environment. In *Pharmacist's Journal,* Issue 12, 1981, a summary discussion of research in this area concluded with the statement, "the release of hydrocyanic acid in the stomach is a possibility but in actuality it is almost impossible for it to happen."

Livestock breeders have used thousands of tons of linseed and linseed flour for years. The *Pharmacist's Journal* piece also commented that there has never been an investigation of acute and chronic toxicity of any other medicine which has been tested over such a long period of time in millions of animals.

## COMPETITION

What competition do omega-3 oils in flaxseed have?

1. **The omega-6 oils.** As previously mentioned, our diets today include high amounts of these oils, actually probably more than at any other time in history. What is needed is to reduce our consumption of these warm-weather oils and increase our consumption of the omega-3 oils.
2. **Fish oils.** There are many arguments over which are better, fish oils that contain omega-3 family members EPA and DHA, or flaxseed oils that contain omega-3 family member LNA. Basically the fish-oil advocates argue that by taking the fish oils, humans are getting their EPA and DHA directly. If LNA is consumed, they reason, there may not be enough enzymes, etc. to change LNA to EPA and DHA. The flax oil people rebut this argument, saying that current research suggests that effecting this change is not a problem and that, if it were, it could be overcome simply by consuming more LNA. Both sides of the argument have distinguished supporters. Perhaps, as Dr. Rudin, author of *The Omega-3 Phenomenon,* suggests, we should consider increasing consumption of both.
3. **Fish.** The traditional dietetic approach is that one will get enough of the right fatty acids found in cold-water fish by eating more of those kinds of fish. While everyone could benefit by consuming more

cold-water fish, one would have to have many fish meals each week, a practice that is not amenable to most people's lifestyle.

4. **Evening primrose oil.** This oil comes from a warm-weather plant that contains over 70 percent omega-6 LA. It also includes about 9 percent GLA (gamma-linolenic acid, no relation to the omega-3 family), which is present in only a few other seeds. The other main nutritional source of GLA is human breast milk.

   GLA is special because it is the product of the body's first biochemical step in the transformation of LA. For a number of reasons—excess cholesterol, excess saturated fats, trans-fatty acids, aging and high sugar consumption—the conversion of LA to GLA does not take place efficiently. Those who support the consumption of evening primrose oil say that it should be consumed in order to assure that proper metabolism of the omega-6 fatty acid LA is taking place even if necessary enzymes are not present.
5. **Saturated fats.** These fats, and the attendant problems related to the amounts in which they are being consumed, are the real competition.

## LOCATING FLAXSEED AND FLAXSEED PRODUCTS

Plain flaxseed, flaxseed (linseed) oil and fortified flaxseed meal can be found in health food stores, drugstores and other outlets. Recipes, which include the use of the omega-3 oils, are available from the producers, and they are included in Dr. Johanna Budwig's book and in Chris Beaman's *Flax Oil Recipe Booklet* (Omega Logic Books, Colorado Springs, Colorado).

### COMPANIES THAT PRODUCE AND MARKET FLAXSEED (LINSEED) PRODUCTS:

Allergy Resources, 6 Main Street, P.O. Box 444, Gussey, Co; tel. 1-719-689-2969.

Omega Nutrition, 1924 Franklin Street, Vancouver, B.C., CANADA V5L1R2; tel. 1-604-253-4677.

Omega Nutrition USA Inc, 6505 Aldrich Road, Bellingham, WA 98226; tel. 1-800-661-3529 or 1-206-384-1238.

Arrowhead Mills, 110 S. Lawton St., Hereford, TX 79045; tel. 1-800-858-4308 or 806-364-0730.

Nutri-Cology, Inc., Allergy Research Group, 400 Preda St., San Leandro, CA 94577; tel. 415-639-4572 or 1-800-545-9660.

Omega-Life, Inc., 15355 Woodbridge Rd., Brookfield, WI 53005; tel. 414-786-2070.

## SUMMARY

The omega-3 and omega-6 oils are two essential fatty acids that work in a complementary fashion to:

- Form the membranes of every one of the billions of cells in our bodies
- Control the way cholesterol works in our systems
- Make up a very large part of the brain's active tissues
- Become prostaglandins, which play key roles in regulating the cardiovascular, immune, digestive and reproductive functions; inflammation and healing; functioning of the brain; and body heat and calorie burning.

Since we know that we are consuming omega-6 oils in great quantities, we need to look at our consumption of omega-3 oils to provide support for all of the above functions. We expect that, because of the types of foods containing omega-3 oils, we simply are not eating the kinds and amounts necessary. All signs point to the conclusion that today, as a nation, we need to consume more omega-3 oils. Since flaxseed has higher levels of omega-3 oils than any other natural product, flaxseed and flaxseed oil should be included in any health-improvement game plan.

In *The Felix Letter,* Clara Felix, coauthor of *The Omega-3 Phenomenon,* advances the need to consume more omega-3 fatty acid foods, noting that this dietary deficit might be the source of some of our present-day health problems.[39]

Her argument is as follows:

- As a nation, we are chronically low in omega-3 fatty acid intake
- Human beings really need to have omega-3 fatty acids
- That omega-3 deficiencies are related to degenerative conditions like heart attacks, arthritis, skin problems, immune system disorders and mental illness.

## SUGGESTED ADDITIONAL READING


Brisson, G. J. *Lipids in Human Nutrition.* Inglewood, New Jersey: Burgess, 1981.

Budwig, J. *Die elementare Funktion der Atmung in ihrer Bezhiehung zu autoxydablen Nahrungstoffen* (The basic functions of cell respiration in its relationship to autooxidizable nutrients—essential fatty acids and sulphurproteins). Freiburg, West Germany: Hyperion Verlag, 1953.

Caliendo, Mary Alice. *Nutrition and Preventive Health Care.* New York: Macmillan Publishing, Inc., 1981.

Erasmus, Udo. *Fats and Oils.* Vancouver, B.C., Canada: Alive Books, 1986.

Fisher, William. *How to Fight Cancer and Win.* Vancouver, B.C., Canada: Alive Books, 1987.

Galland, Leo and Buchman, Dian Dincin. *Superimmunity for Kids.* New York: E. P. Dutton, 1988.

Garrison, Robert H., Jr. and Somer, Elizabeth. *The Nutrition Desk Reference.* New Canaan, Connecticut: Keats Publishing, Inc., 1985.

Gold, Robert and Rose-Gold, Kerry. *The Good Fat Diet.* New York: Bantam Books, 1987.

Horrobin, D. F. *Essential Fatty Acids, a Review.* In Horrobin, D. F. (ed.), *Clinical Uses of Essential Fatty Acids.* London, England: Eden Press, 1982.

Mead, J. F., and Fulco, A. J. *The Unsaturated and Polyunsaturated Fatty Acids in Health and Disease.* Springfield, Illinois: Charles C Thomas, 1976.

Niazi, S. K. *The Omega Connection.* Westchester, Illinois: Esquire Books, Inc., 1988.

Rudin, Donald O., and Felix, Clara. *The Omega-3 Phenomenon: The Nutrition Breakthrough of the '80s.* New York: Rawson Associates, 1987.

Sinclair, H. M. *Essential Fatty Acids.* London, England: Butterworths, 1958.

Werbach, Melvyn R. *Nutritional Influences on Illness.* New Canaan, Connecticut: Keats Publishing, Inc., 1988.

## REFERENCES

1. Califano, J. A. What's wrong with U.S. health care? *Washington Post,* June 26, 1977.
2. Caliendo, M. A. *Nutrition and Preventive Health Care* (New York: Macmillan Publishing Co., Inc., 1981), 1.
3. U.S. Department of Health, Education and Welfare. *Ten-State Survey, 1968–70,* Publ. No. (HSM) 72–8134. Washington, D. C.: Government Printing Office, 1972.
4. National Center for Health Statistics. *Preliminary Findings of the First Health and Nutrition Examination Survey, 1971–72.* Washington, D. C.: Government Printing Office, January 1974.
5. U.S. Senate Select Committee on Nutrition and Human Needs. *Dietary Goals for the United States,* Second Edition. Washington, D. C.: Government Printing Office, December 1977.
6. Belloc, N. B., and Breslow, L. Relationship of physical health status and health practices. *Prev. Med.* 1 (1972): 409.
7. Popkin, B. Economic benefits from the elimination of hunger in America. *Public Policy 20* (1972): 133.
8. Weir, C. E. *Benefits from Human Nutrition Research.* Washington, D. C.: U. S. Department of Agriculture, Science and Education Staff, 1971.
9. Winikoff, B. In U.S. Senate Select Committee on Nutrition and Human Needs, *Diet Related to Killer Diseases.* Washington, D. C.: Government Printing Office, July 27–28, 1976.
10. Erasmus, U. *Fats and Oils* (Vancouver: Alive Books, 1986), 80, 319.
11. Rudin, D. O., and Felix, C. *The Omega-3 Phenomenon* (New York: Rawson Associates, 1987), 8.
12. Ibid.
13. Hamilton, E. M. N., *et al. Nutrition, Concepts and Controversies* (St. Paul, Minnesota: West Publishing, 1988), 118.
14. Straight talk about fats and your health. Petaluma, Calif.: Spectrum Naturals, 1988.
15. Stitt, P. *Efficacy of Feeding Flax to Humans and Other Animals.* Address to the Flax Research Priorities Conference of the Flax Council of Canada, March 21–22, 1988.

16. Hanley, G. *Growing Flax* (Saskatchewan, Saskatchewan Agricultural Fund, 1988), 2.
17. Bland, J. S. The changing nature of dietary fats and oils. *Let's Live,* November 1987, 68–69.
18. Sinclair, H. M. Valedictory Address. *Prog. Fd. Nutr. Sci.* 4 (1980): 131–134.
19. Erasmus, *Fats and Oils,* 231.
20. Budwig, J. *Die elementäre Funktion der Atmung in ihrer Beziehung zu autoxydablen Nahrungstoffen* (Freiburg, German Federal Republic: Hyperion Verlag, 1953), 14.
21. Hildenbrand, G. Editor. Fats that heal, fats that kill. *Healing Newsletter* NL22 and 23 (Bonita, California: Gerson Institute, 1988):2.
22. Rudin, D. O., *The Omega-3 Phenomenon,* 15–22.
23. Dyerberg, J., Bang, H. O., and Hjorne, N. Fatty acid composition of plasma lipids in Greenland Eskimos. *Am. J. Clin. Nutr.* 28 (1975): 958–966.
24. Stitt, P. Nutritional importance of flax. *Flax Growers Newsletter* November 1986: 13.
25. Ibid.
26. Ibid.
27. Ibid.
28. Ibid. 14.
29. Fisher, W. L. *How to Fight Cancer and Win* (Vancouver: Alive Books, 1987), 128.
30. Ibid., 131.
31. Ibid., 128.
32. Cunnane, S. *Preliminary Research on the Nutritional Effects of Flax in the Treatment of Cardiovascular Disease.* Address to the Flax Research Priorities Conference of the Flax Council of Canada, March 21–22, 1988.
33. Dickinson, A. R. P. Scherer Survey of Health and Nutrition Literature. *Omega-3 Fatty Acids Review* VIII, no. 6 (June 1988).
34. Ibid.
35. See note 32 above.
36. Aldercreutz, H. Does fiber-rich food containing lignin precursors protect against both colon and breast cancer? An extension of the "Fiber Hypothesis." *Gastroenterology* 4, no. 86 (1984): 761–766.
37. See note 15 above.
38. Ibid.
39. Felix, C. Classic pellagra. *The Felix Letter* (Berkeley, Cal. 1988), 2.

# NUTRITION UPDATE: FATS

Which is better: margarine or butter, safflower oil or olive oil? Are avocados and nuts "bad" foods? Can I relax when a product label promises 100% vegetable oil, even if it's partially hydrogenated?

There is probably no nutrition topic so fraught with confusion and misunderstanding than the world of fats and oils. New research is emerging every day, but not all of it comes up with the same answers. To compound the problem, food manufacturers have altered natural vegetable oils in ways that diminish rather than enhance health and then confuse consumers with outrageous claims and misleading labels. The new labeling laws may help a little.

The paradox is this: The typical meat-eating, fast-food loving, ice cream-savoring American overconsumes fat to an alarming degree, which leads not only to overweight, but to an increased risk of heart disease, cancer, diabetes, hypertension and other lifestyle-induced ailments. At the same time, however, most Americans may be deficient in the specific fats that their bodies need.

Not all fats are bad fats. In fact, a certain kind of fat is vital to a healthy diet. Fat is an essential nutrient, just as protein is. These "essential" fats cannot be manufactured by the body; they must be provided in the foods we eat.

Thus, the fat fanatic who tries to remove every last glob of fat from his diet may have gone too far to the other extreme. The only time a severely fat-restricted diet (10% or less of calories) makes sense is if one is trying to reverse a serious medical condition such as obesity, heart disease or cancer.

For the rest of us, avocados and nuts can have an honorable place in a healthy whole foods diet. They certainly don't deserve to be lumped together, as many dietary guidelines do, with other fatty no-nos like hot dogs, pastrami, and ice cream, whose dietary impact is purely negative. In a study reported in the *American Journal of Clinical Nutrition* (October 1992) it was found that women who supplemented their otherwise low-fat diets with avocados were more likely to lower their cholesterol levels, maintain a high HDL ("good" cholesterol) level, and stick with their diet than women on a standard low-fat diet. Avocados are second only to olive oil as a rich source of health-promoting mono-unsaturated fat.

Similar results were found in a study reported in the *Archives of Internal Medicine* (July 1992) about nuts and coronary heart disease. This was an epidemiological study of diet and heart disease prevalence among 31,208 Seventh-Day Adventists. In correlating the intakes of cheese, nuts, beef, fish, coffee, bread, fruit, and legumes with heart disease, the study found that nuts and whole wheat bread consistently showed a statistically significant relationship between high intake and low heart disease incidence. In addition to the mono-unsaturated oil in the nuts, both contain substantial amounts of heart-healthy vitamin E.

Which other foods contain these essential fats? Not the saturated animal fats we are overconsuming, nor, as research continues to show, the margarine or other hydrogenated or processed oils. The important health-giving unsaturated oils are found in leafy green vegetables, whole grains, seeds, nuts, and fish.

## GONE BAD

Fats in the American diet have been chemically altered beyond recognition. Commercially processed vegetable oils, oils that have been hydrogenated, extracted with chemical solvents, bleached, purified, heated to high temperatures and turned into margarine or other partially hydrogenated vegetable oils are good fats turned bad.

To turn an oil such as corn or safflower into a solid such as margarine, a chemical process called hydrogenation must take place. This process turns the natural or "cis fat" into a man-made partially hydrogenated or "trans fat." These trans fats are anti-nutrients. They block the development of prostaglandins, hormone-like substances that are vital in regulating not only the cardiovascular system, but the reproductive system, the central nervous system and the immune system. Some researchers believe that the onset of any disease can be attributed to a prostaglandin imbalance. Research continues to show that margarine clogs arteries as relentlessly as saturated fat does and is linked with tumor growth in animals.

Thus, in the context of a low-fat diet, a diet that derives 20 to 25% of its calories from fat and 65% of its calories from whole grains, vegetables, and fruits, a tablespoon of sweet butter each day can do no harm. For cooking and salads, choose olive or canola oils. Canola oil is a good source of the essential omega-3 oils which are also found in salmon and other fatty cold-water ocean fish, as well as in the leaves of green, leafy vegetables (particularly purslane, sea vegetables and spinach), soybeans, flax and pumpkin seeds. Research has shown that these health-promoting oils can lower triglyceride levels, inhibit free radical development, tame the inflammatory response, prevent blood clotting, and lower LDL (bad) cholesterol.

Above all, read labels and avoid foods prepared with hydrogenated or partially hydrogenated oils. It is not only the quantity of fats and oils we must pay attention to, but the kinds of fats and oils.

PHYLLIS HERMAN, M.S., C.N.S.

# OLIVE OIL

*Mediterranean Green Gold*

••

Jean Barilla, M.S.

MEDITERRANEAN GREEN GOLD

Over 6,000 years ago, the olive tree was first cultivated in the Mediterranean countries. Since the Bronze Age, olive oil has been the basic cooking oil and a cornerstone of the economy. It was used as a fuel, in cosmetics and soaps, during religious ceremonies and, most importantly, as a therapeutic agent. Hippocrates, the most celebrated physician of ancient times (400 BC) recommend olive oil for curing ulcers, cholera, gall bladder problems and muscular pains. Scientific research has since substantiated what the ancient healers knew—that olive oil was important in the prevention and treatment of cardiovascular diseases, some forms of cancer, and inflammatory conditions such as arthritis, and is necessary for normal cellular function.

## WHAT'S IN IT FOR YOU?

The key to obtaining the full health benefits of olive oil, is that it must be unrefined or virgin. The whole, ripe, undamaged olive fruit must be pressed, without heat, to yield a liquid where more than 80 percent of the fatty acids are beneficial to health.

Olive oil contains mainly nonessential monounsaturated fatty acids

(MUFAs) with small amounts of the essential fatty acids, linoleic and alpha-linolenic acids.

> MUFAs in olive oil:
>
> Linoleic acid (omega-6)—3.5 percent to 20 percent (average 10 percent)
> Alpha-linolenic (omega-3)—0.1 percent to 6 percent
> Oleic acid (omega-9)—63 percent to 83 percent (average 75 percent)
> Palmitoleic acid (omega-7)—0.5 percent to 3 percent (average 2 percent)

Oleic acid increases the incorporation of omega-3 fatty acids in cell membranes, thus maintaining the fluidity and function of this cell structure. It also decreases the oxidation of LDL, reducing its atherogenic potential (see below).

Olive oil also contains saturated fatty acids: palmitic acid ranges from 7.5 percent to 18 percent (average 10 percent). Palmitic acid is known to raise cholesterol levels, yet olive oil *protects* arteries rather than damaging them. The amount of stearic acid, which neither raises nor lowers cholesterol levels is about 2 percent.

There are several minor, but important, components in olive oil including the antioxidants beta-carotene and tocopherols (vitamin E family). Chlorophyll, rich in magnesium, is found in unrefined green oils such as olive, hemp, pumpkin and avocado. Patients with cardiovascular disease are often magnesium deficient. Squalene is another component. This substance helps deliver oxygen to tissues, especially those short of oxygen. It also increases heart activity, dilates blood vessels and inhibits atherosclerosis. Olive oil also contains phytosterols such as beta-sitosterol. These compounds protect against cholesterol absorption from foods, thus lowering cholesterol levels. Polyphenols, plant compounds with antioxidant abilities, help stabilize the oil.

## FROM PUFAs TO MUFAs AND THEN SOME

In the 1960s, researchers noted that monounsaturated fatty acids (MUFAs) and carbohydrates did not affect plasma cholesterol levels. Polyunsaturated fatty acids (PUFAs) were found to lower total plasma cholesterol and LDL cholesterol (the "bad" cholesterol). So, it was recommended that PUFAs replace saturated fatty acids in the diet. However, that wasn't the whole story. PUFAs were also found to lower HDL cholesterol (the "good" cholesterol) and high intake was implicated in increasing susceptibility to gallstones and cancer that was induced by chemical substances.

Later studies found that both MUFA or PUFA decreased LDL. Because of the lack of evidence of the safety of high PUFA diets, and the negative effect on HDL, MUFAs were instead recommended to replace dietary saturated fatty acids. Although there was subsequent data to indicate that a diet balanced in amounts of MUFA and PUFA would have similar beneficial effects, other effects of MUFAs tipped the scales in favor of increasing dietary MUFAs. Among these findings was the fact that plasma cholesterol levels are lower in countries with a high content of oleic acid (the major fatty acid in olive oil), present in the diet. MUFAs were found to be better for non-insulin-dependent diabetics than low-fat, high-carbohydrate diets since there is also a triglyceride-lowering effect. Blood pressure-lowering effects were also found with diets high in oleic acid.

Diets high in MUFAs also protect LDL from oxidation, the process that makes LDL become "bad." LDL cholesterol itself is not "bad." When it is not protected by antioxidants such as vitamin E and MUFAs, however, it becomes oxidized and contributes to atherosclerosis. When olive oil is added to the diet it enriches the LDL molecule with oleic acid and sitosterol, making the LDL more resistant to oxidation.

In addition to heart disease, research is now being conducted on the effects of olive oil consumption on rheumatoid arthritis. It was found that patients with the disease consumed significantly less olive oil (and fish oil) than individuals who had less of these nutrients in their diets. In the U.S., a study is now being conducted by The National Arthritis Foundation, to determine the effects of olive oil supplementation on patients with arthritis.

## THE MEDITERRANEAN DIET

There is evidence that a so-called Mediterranean diet has important and beneficial effects on the rate of occurrence of coronary heart disease (CHD) and other disease states. Olive oil is the backbone of the Mediterranean diet, providing a larger number of calories than any other single food. Starting in the 1950s, Dr. A. Keys and colleagues followed 12,000 middle-aged men in seven different countries for 30 years. One of the most significant results of the study was that mortality rates were lower for Greek men than for northern European, American and Japanese groups. The difference was especially striking for CHD.

In the early 1980s researchers studied the dietary intake of 14 Mediterranean countries (Portugal, Spain, France, Italy, Yugoslavia, Greece, Malta, Israel, Libya, Algeria, Tunisia, Turkey, Egypt, and Morocco) and found a common nutritional profile (perhaps the only time that these countries were in agreement with each other in any way). Diets in these countries were characterized by a low intake of saturated fat, moderate intake of total fat, mainly monounsaturated (olive oil), and high intake of complex carbohydrates.

## FOLLOW THE GREEKS

The Greek version of the Mediterranean diet was especially considered optimal because life expectancy in Greece was higher than in the U.S., and heart disease and total cancers were less prevalent. The traditional Greek diet is low in saturated fat, high in monounsaturated fat (namely olive oil), high in complex carbohydrates from grains and legumes, and high in fiber—mostly from vegetables and fruits. The high content of fresh fruits and vegetables and cereal and liberal use of olive oil ensures a high intake of beta-carotene, vitamin C, tocopherols, many minerals and other phytonutrients (plant-based nutrients) such as polyphenols and proanthocyanadins. Moderate intake of wine was also considered a positive factor. Greeks also eat more fish and less meat and fewer eggs than U.S. populations.

There are few factors other than diet that can explain the remarkable health advantages enjoyed by Greek men (and to a lesser extent, women) in the 1960s and 1970s. The frequency and intensity of smoking by Greek men are among the highest in the world, intentional physical exercise is rarely practiced in Greece (much of the population is rural, however, and individuals are not usually sedentary), and there are no nation-wide programs for early detection and effective treatment of high blood pressure. The advantage decreases, however, as Greeks change their traditional diet and food culture.

During the past ten years, several research findings have increased the credibility of the effect of diet on CHD in Greeks. Studies have determined that high levels of HDL cholesterol, moderate drinking of alcoholic beverages, intake of fiber and fruit and vegetables all decrease the risk of CHD. Also, strong evidence that partially hydrogenated vegetable fats (margarine and vegetable shortening) increase CHD, and the fact that Greeks eat very little margarine, provide further evidence on a dietary cause and effect.

Although other factors such as the relaxing psychological environment, the stress-releasing habit of taking afternoon siestas, preservation of the extended family structure, and even mild climatic conditions may complement the beneficial effects of the traditional diet, the Greek diet is still the central factor in lowering the risk of CHD. Although the average Greek obtains 40 percent of dietary calories from fat, considerably above the "under 30 percent level" recommended in the U.S., this population has had and still has one of the longest life expectancies of all nationalities.

Other studies, evaluating the diet of Greek women, found that higher intakes of vegetables and fruits correlated with significant reduction in breast cancer risk. There was also evidence that olive oil consumption reduced breast cancer, while margarine was associated with an elevated risk for the disease. In another study on diet and breast cancer in Spain, higher consumption of olive oil was significantly related to a lower risk of breast cancer.

## FOOD PYRAMID OR GREEK COLUMN?

Many countries have developed their own food guides or "pyramids." A common theme for these guidelines is recommendation of lower fat, saturated fat and cholesterol; less salt and sugar; and more fresh fruits and vegetables. In each country, the composition of the pyramid is based on that country's traditional diet. The Mexican (or Mayan) pyramid is based on fruits, vegetables and whole grains. Oriental-type guidelines are based on rice and vegetables. Only the U.S. Department of Agriculture's food guide pyramid has grains as the base, or major dietary platform.

According to Dr. Artemis P. Simopoulos, President of The Center for Genetics, Nutrition and Health, grains are newcomers to our diet from an evolutionary viewpoint. Grains only became a staple in our diets about 10,000 years ago. The U.S. pyramid is a high-carbohydrate/low-fat diet, with not enough emphasis on fruits and vegetables.

Diets high in carbohydrates elevate triglycerides, another contributing factor to heart disease. Our ancestors ate diets high in fruits and vegetables that contained a high content of antioxidant vitamins (vitamins E, C, beta-carotene) and more calcium, folate and fiber. Antioxidants are known to decrease the risk of heart disease, cancer, and prevent or treat many other major diseases (see The Nutrition Superbook Volume I, *The Antioxidants*).

The most important criticism of the U.S. food pyramid is that it does not distinguish among the various fatty acids, such as trans fatty acids and omega-3 and omega-6 polyunsaturated fatty acids. It does not emphasize the beneficial effects of olive oil in raising HDL cholesterol or in protecting LDL cholesterol from oxidation.

While the Greek diet is high in monounsaturates, the American diet is high in polyunsaturated fatty acids, from vegetable oils rich in omega-6 fatty acids. Such a diet is low in omega-3 fatty acids, creating imbalances that lead to increased tendency to inflammatory and thrombotic conditions. As use of omega-6 fatty acids increases, prostaglandins and leukotrienes that promote constriction of blood vessels and clotting are made.

Dr. Simopoulos' model for an ideal diet, based on genetic variation and nutrition, is the "Greek Column." It is based on human evolution and on the food that people of the Mediterranean region ate before 1960, with perhaps more fish and poultry. Olive oil is the main cooking oil while other vegetable oils and hydrogenated oils are excluded. At the base of the column are foods that can be easily incorporated in any meal: olive oil, lemon, vinegar, olives. These foods are rich in antioxidant vitamins and minerals and have a natural balance of omega-6 and omega-3 fatty acids.

There is no limit to how much oil to eat as long as body weight levels are normal. Completing the base of the column are: bread, cheese, yogurt, fruits and fruit juices, nuts, garlic, onions, vegetables, herbs, spices, pasta, rice, potatoes; and water and wine. Above these basic foods, to be consumed in lesser amounts, are legumes, fish, and poultry. Meat and eggs are part of a main meal once a week each. There is no place for margarines and other artificial foods. Sweets are eaten rarely or on special occasions, as is true for soft drinks and hard liquor.

## SUMMARY

As we are being told to reduce our fat intake to less than 30 percent of calories, in order to avoid the ravages of heart disease and various kinds of cancer, the research discussed above is demonstrating that it is possible to eat just as much fat as ever, yet remain protected

> FIGURE OUT THE FAT—FAST
>
> There's a simple calculation that can help you determine the percentage of calories that come from fat in any packaged food, from crackers to frozen entrees. You just need to know the amount of fat and the number of calories per serving—information found on any standard nutrition label.
>
> Here's an example using a frozen Chinese dinner that has 20 grams of fat and 340 calories per serving.
>
> First multiply the number of grams of fat (20) by the number of calories per gram (1 gram equals 9 calories). The total number of calories derived from fat per serving is 180.
>
> Then divide the number of fat calories (180) by the calories (340) and multiply by 100. (A calculator comes in handy here.)
>
> The answer: 53% of the calories in this dinner comes from fat. The verdict: Put it back in the store's freezer.

from the chronic diseases that plague so many of us during the last 10 to 20 years of our lives. The key to eating fats and oils, as demonstrated in this book, is knowing what type to eat.

Many of would be more pleased to follow diets that include more fat than the U.S. Dietary Guidelines diet, with its "lean" instructions for choosing a diet low in fat. The composition of fatty acids in olive oil places it at the top of the list when it comes to taste and good health.

This chapter contains information that will be included in the Keats Good Health Guide, *Olive Oil Miracle,* by Jean Barilla, M.S., to be published later this year.

## BIBLIOGRAPHY

Pagnan, A., Bonanome, A. Position statement: Monounsaturated fatty acids in human nutrition. *J Amer Coll Nutr.* 1992;11 (S) :79S-81S.

Berry, E. M., *et al.* Effects of diets rich in monounsaturated fatty acids on plasma lipoproteins—the Jerusalem Nutrition Study. III Monounsaturated fatty acids vs. carbohydrates. *Am J Clin Nutr.* 1992;56:394-403.

Aviram, M. Eias, K. Dietary olive oil reduces low-density lipoprotein uptake by macrophages and decreases the susceptibility of the lipoprotein to undergo lipid peroxidation. *Annals of Nutr & Metab.* 1993;37(2):75-84.

Barilla, J. *Olive Oil Miracle.* Keats Publishing, Inc. New Canaan, Connecticut, in press.

Trichopoulou, A., Lagiou, P., Trichopoulos, D. Traditional Greek diet and coronary heart disease. *J Cardiovasc Risk.* 1994;1:9-15.

Trichopoulou A., *et al.* Consumption of olive oil and specific food groups in relation to breast cancer risk in Greece. *J Natl Cancer Inst.* 1995;87(2):110-116.

Martin-Moreno, J. M. *et al.* Dietary fat, olive oil intake and breast cancer risk. *Int. J Cancer* 1994;58(6):774-780.

Simopoulos, A. P. The Mediterranean food guide. Greek column rather than an Egyptian pyramid. *Nutrition Today.* 1995;30(2):54-61.

Linos, A., *et al.* The effect of olive oil and fish consumption on rheumatoid arthritis—a case control study. *Scand, J. Rheum.* 1991;20(6):419-426.

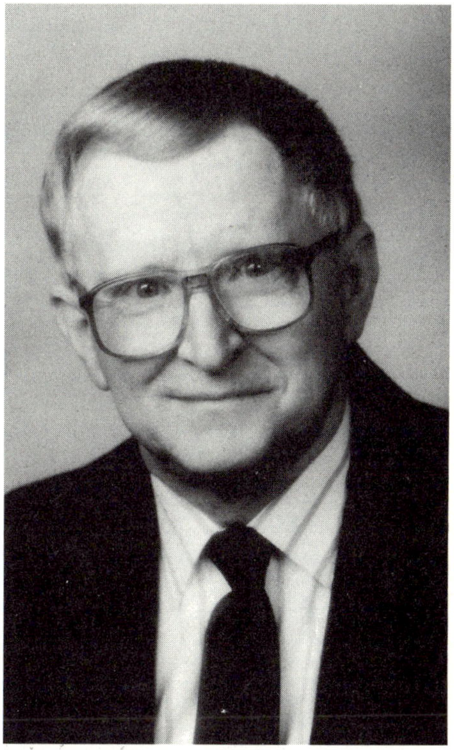

Richard A. Passwater, Ph.D. (EPA-Marine Lipids, Fish Oils, Evening Primrose Oil, Lipoic Acid) a noted biochemist, has taken research out of the laboratory and put it in the hands of readers worldwide; he is credited with popularizing the term "supernutrition."

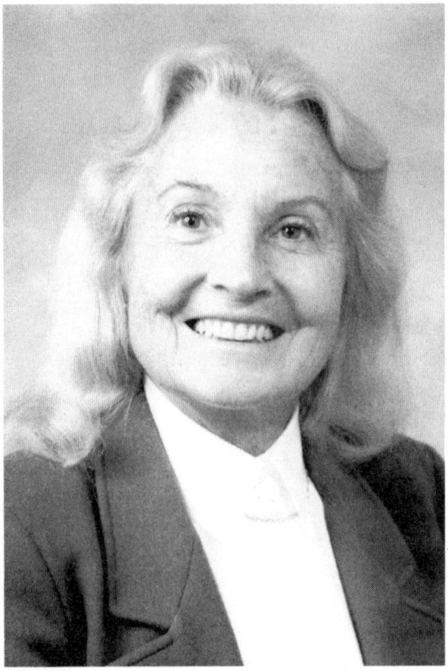

**Ingeborg M. Johnston** (Flaxseed [Linseed] Oil and the Power of Omega-3, with James R. Johnston, Ph.D.) is a Certified Nutritionist and Registered Nurse. She and her husband are involved in education of Certified Nutritionists for the National Institute of Nutritional Education.

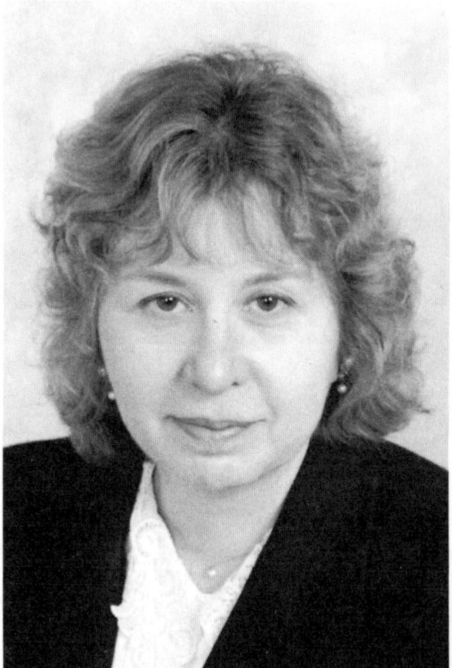

**Jean Barilla, M.S.** (Olive Oil-Mediterranean Green Gold and series editor for *The Nutrition Superbooks*) is a medical writer whose writing appears in medical journals, medical-legal textbooks, magazines and newspapers. Jean writes a medical newsletter for physicians and hosts a radio health talk show.

His commitment to nutrition education for the public and for health professionals has put **Jeffrey Bland, Ph.D.** (Choline, Lecithin and Inositol; Octacosanol, Carnitine and Taurine) in the national spotlight as an author, lecturer and president of his own health communication firm.

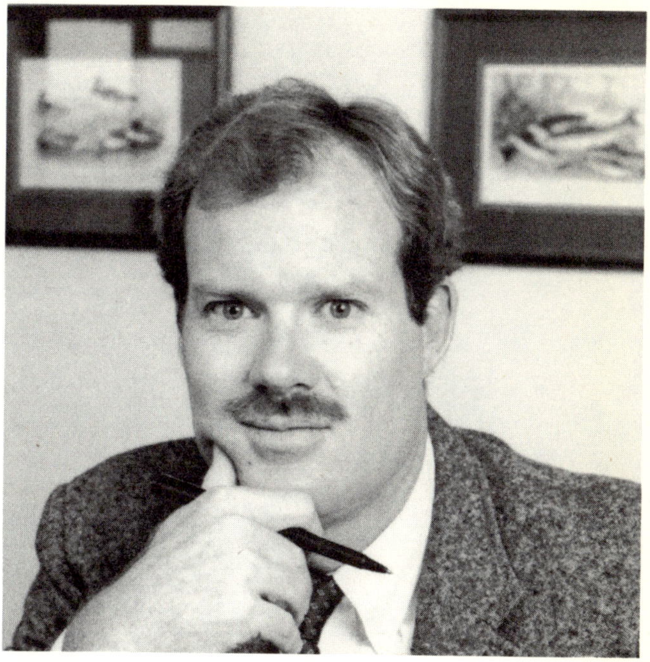

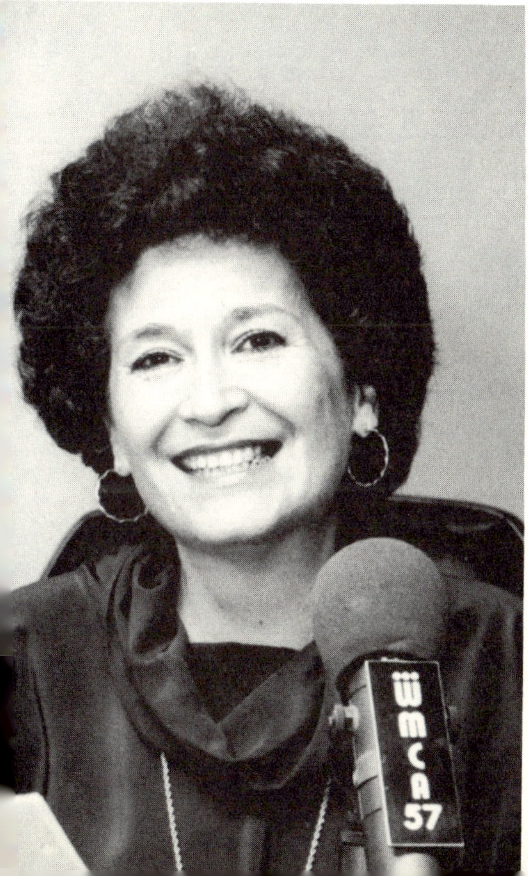


**Betty Kamen, Ph.D.** (Sesame) is a well-known author and consumer health advocate. She and her husband, Si Kamen, have produced nationally recognized health-related TV shows and filmstrips.

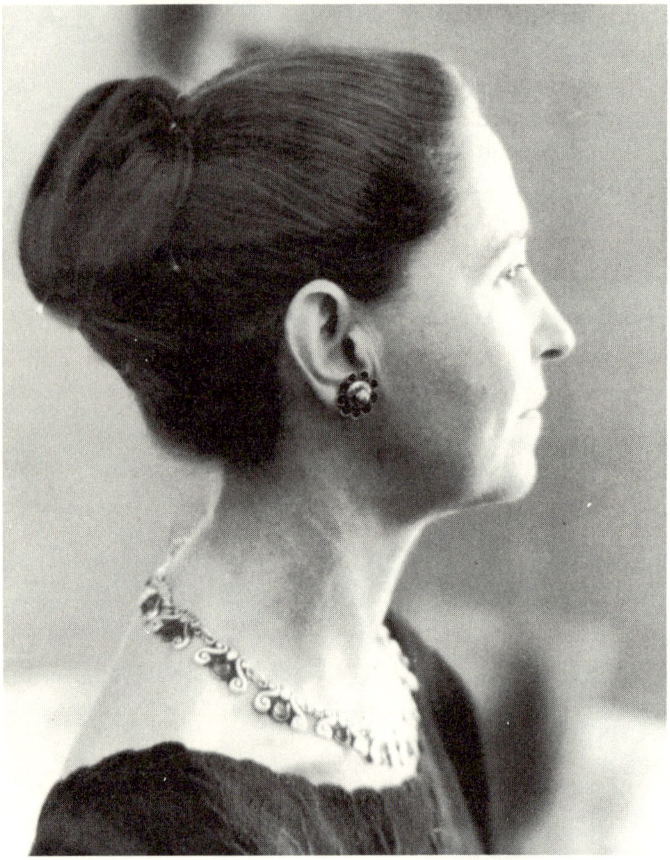

One of America's foremost food experts and consumer advocates, **Beatrice Trum Hunter** (Brewer's Yeast, Wheat Germ and Other High Power Foods) lectures widely and is food editor of *Consumers' Research Magazine.*

# PART THREE

# THE FAT PARTNERS

# CHOLINE, LECITHIN AND INOSITOL

JEFFREY BLAND, PH.D.

EXCITING DISCOVERIES

The health maverick in each of us—the one that governs those unique needs which do not conform to "normal" standards—can now be satisfied through this family of food "accessories": dietary supplements of lecithin, if you can't make enough yourself, to conquer cholesterol and aid memory; or inositol, to help the liver manage fat and help nerves grow. These nutrients possess powerful therapeutic value for specific individuals and occupy an exciting area in nutritional development.

## THE ACCESSORY NUTRIENTS IN HEALTH PROMOTION

The role that vitamins and minerals play in human nutrition has been established through years of clinical and biochemical research. Their important function in activating specific enzymes and serving as cellular protective agents is well established, and the therapeutic usefulness of vitamin and mineral factors when given in doses above that of the Recommended Dietary Allowances is receiving greater and greater attention.

There is another class of nutrients which are concentrated from food and are now receiving equal attention. These are not members of the essential nutrient family, but rather are termed "accessory food factors." Accessory food factors and essential vitamins or minerals are distinguished by important recognizable differences.

An essential nutrient is a substance, such as vitamin B1 (thiamine) or vitamin B2 (riboflavin), or vitamin C (ascorbic acid), which cannot be manufactured within the human body and must be obtained from the diet where another plant or animal has produced it. Essential nutrients must be consumed in the human diet in adequate amounts to meet the needs of health promotion.

A few essential nutrients fall outside of this rigorous definition and still are considered to be vitamin factors. An example is vitamin D, which can be manufactured in a person's body by exposure to full-spectrum sunlight, or vitamin B12 which can be partially manufactured by bacteria in the gastrointestinal tract, or vitamin B3 (niacin) which can be partly manufactured in the liver from dietary tryptophan, although not at levels adequate to meet the needs of most healthy people.

These agents are considered to be vitamin factors since their ability to be manufactured in the human body is inadequate for prevention of known vitamin deficiency diseases, such as pernicious anemia with vitamin B12 or pellagra with vitamin B3, and therefore must be obtained from the diet.

The accessory food factors, on the other hand, are materials which are manufactured within the human body, at levels that would be considered "adequate" for most individuals. The important distinction is that many of these accessory metabolites native to the human body may not be manufactured at *optimal* levels for the promotion of health, and therefore may be more useful when taken in the diet or as a food supplement. This frames the basic concept of the therapeutic use of accessory food factors in clinical nutrition. Any person may require one or more of these accessory food factors to be consumed in greater amounts than the average diet provides because of his or her unique health or genetic state.

The list of nutrients which may possess powerful therapeutic value when given in enhanced doses to specific individuals is one of the most exciting areas of clinical nutrition. A partial list of such factors is shown below:

| Representative Accessory Nutrients |
|---|
| Beta-carotene |
| Bioflavonoids |
| Carnitine |
| Choline (lecithin) |
| Dietary fibers |
| Dimethylglycine |
| Garlic concentrate |
| Inositol |
| Octacosanol |
| Saponins |
| Specific amino acids |
| Specific oil concentrates (i.e., marine lipids such as EPA) |
| Taurine |
| Vegetable gums |
| Xanthophylls |

To illustrate the principle of the use of a therapeutic food factor in clinical nutrition one need only look at a condition such as phenylketonuria. Phenylketonuria is a genetic condition in which an infant is born without the ability to metabolize the amino acid phenylalanine properly in the diet. This amino acid comes from dietary protein. When it cannot be properly metabolized, it builds up in the body and causes mental retardation.

Traditionally, the treatment of this condition has been to put the infant on a diet low in phenylalanine. However, investigators have suggested that phenylketonuria may be better treated by administering augmented supplies of the amino acid tyrosine, made from phenylalanine, which may be deficient due to a metabolic block. In clinical studies, when tyrosine was administered to infants who had phenylketonuria in the absence of a phenylalanine restricted diet, their IQ and performance actually were better than when the infants had been placed on a phenylalanine-restricted diet.[1] This indicates that possibly for these individuals the symptoms of retardation are really a result of tyrosine deficiency, and for them tyrosine becomes an essential amino acid that must be acquired through diet or supplements. In such cases an accessory food factor becomes an essential nutrient. This is called the *justification hypothesis,* which states that certain nutrients usually manufactured in the individual's own body may be essential in certain individuals because of their genetic limitation in the ability to manufacture the substance in adequate quantities.[2]

The proposal of Dr. Roger Williams some fifty years ago of biochemical individuality is the theme upon which this particular concept is based. Dr. Williams suggested that genetotrophic diseases are diseases that can be ameliorated or prevented by augmenting the supply of one or more constituents within food, based upon the individual's genetic uniqueness.[3]

Specific health or medical conditions may also require an enhanced intake of one of the accessory food factors. The recognition of specific biochemical needs for these accessory food factors opened the door for a whole new field of clinical nutrition.

This chapter will discuss the clinical usefulness of three such accessory food factors which represent the general field. The future for the use of these substances is very rich, and as we learn more about food concentrates and the principles within them, we begin to recognize the panoramic clinical utility of the accessory food factors.

Essential oils such as evening primrose oil and fish oil from cold water fish (such as mackerel and salmon) providing omega-3 EPA have shown usefulness in enhancing immune function and reducing blood cholesterol and the risk of heart disease.[4,5] These two additional examples of accessory food factors have also been demonstrated to have therapeutic benefit in controlled human studies.

## CHOLINE AND LECITHIN

### DIETARY SOURCES AND THE DIFFERENCE BETWEEN CHOLINE AND LECITHIN

Choline is a well recognized member of the B-complex vitamin family; however, dietary deficiency of choline has only been demonstrated to produce liver problems in animals, and no acute deficiency has been seen in humans. This is in part a result of the fact that choline can be manufactured in the human body and therefore is not truly an essential nutrient, but rather a member of the accessory food factor family.[6]

Choline has been used therapeutically in human studies to prevent alcoholic cirrhosis and liver damage, but with varying success.[7] In the body, choline is utilized as a substance from which phosphatidylcholine, which is called lecithin, is manufactured. As seen in Figure 1, lecithin is made up of a glycerol backbone with two fatty acids and a phosphatidylcholine residue which are combined chemically. In the lecithin molecule the fatty acids can either be of the saturated or unsaturated fatty acid families. The more highly saturated lecithins come from animal sources and are solid at room temperature, whereas the more unsaturated lecithins are generally from vegetable origin and are liquid at room temperature. The body manufactures lecithin in the liver, which it utilizes for the formation of proper bile. This lecithin is manufactured from choline that comes from both the diet and the body's own manufacturing process.

The concentration of choline in the body and the blood depends upon dietary choline intake. Dietary lecithin also elevates tissue and serum choline levels. Foods such as eggs, liver, soybeans and peanuts have the highest dietary concentration of choline. Once the dietary lecithin has been ingested, it is broken down in the intestinal tract to substances which are absorbed into the blood and then remade into lecithin in the liver. A food-ingested dose of choline at the level of 0.3 grams per kilogram of body weight will increase the blood level

FIGURE 1
THE LECITHIN MOLECULE

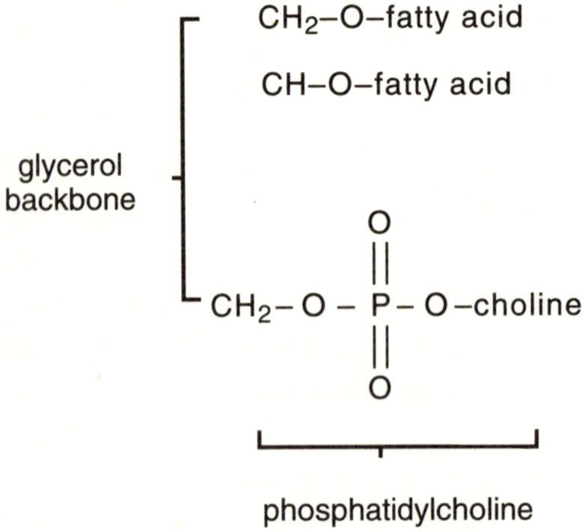


of choline by 400 percent, and this will last for twelve hours.[8] The normal dietary intake of choline is approximately 300 mg a day, coming from a wide variety of foods. Lecithin has been utilized as a dietary source of choline for certain therapeutic trials, but it should be recalled that commercial lecithin has a wide variety of compositions, as it relates to their choline content. The highly concentrated and purified lecithins, in which the composition is greater than 30 percent phosphatidylcholine, will supply the highest amounts of choline and lead to the greatest blood elevations of choline after oral administration.

## USE OF LECITHIN IN HUMAN BIOCHEMISTRY

Choline and lecithin are absorbed in the upper intestine and seem to be transmitted to the blood by passive diffusion, meaning the higher the amount in the diet, the more will appear in the blood. One of the major problems in utilizing choline in large doses as a supplement is that part of it is broken down in the intestines to a substance called trimethylamine, which has the odor of rotten fish. The intestinal bacteria manufacture trimethylamine from high levels of dietary choline and the individual takes on a characteristic odor as a result of the choline therapy. It has been found that the use of lecithin in high levels will deliver to the blood high levels of choline, but will not be cleaved in the intestinal tract to trimethylamine, so the unpleasant fishy odor is avoided.

There are a number of tissues which have been shown to utilize the high blood levels of choline in the manufacture of specific substances such as lecithin or acetylcholine. (Acetylcholine is secreted at the nerve junctions helping to transport messages across nerve junctions, to ensure proper nervous system function.[9] It is a well-known member of the neurotransmitter family.) The tissues which use choline include the brain, kidney, liver and spleen. Three tissues—the liver, the testes and the heart—are known to be able to synthesize choline, and this is why it is not generally considered an essential nutrient. However, these three organs are capable of making only about 15 percent of the daily need, and therefore if a diet does not contain adequate levels of choline or lecithin, then subtle signs of undernutrition can appear. The major role of choline, once absorbed in the body and transported in the blood to the tissues that need it, is as a stimulator of the synthesis of lecithin as a raw material from which acetylcholine is synthesized. Choline also functions as a member of the lipotrophic vitamin family involved in methyl donation in the conversion to another member of this lipotrophic family, betaine.

The therapeutic usefulness of lecithin and choline is to a great extent related to their readiness to be converted to acetylcholine.

## CHOLINE IN FETAL DEVELOPMENT AND THE NEWBORN

It has been found that newborns have extremely high choline content in their blood, which seems to be necessary for the manufacture of the nervous system insulator called myelin, and for the synthesis of the membranes of many cells within the nervous system and brain.[10] Deficiencies of choline in the newborn or the fetus may produce profound developmental abnormalities related to the nervous system. Human milk, which is 3.8 percent fat, as compared to cow's milk, which is 3 to 5 percent fat, has much higher levels of lecithin than cow's milk. These lecithins are used by the developing fetus for the manufacture of a long surfactant material which prevents infection and other lung disorders once the fetus has been delivered. Low manufacture of this lung surfactant material can lead to respiratory distress in the infant, one of the major neonatal problems, particularly in premature birth. Proper transport of choline across the placental barrier from the mother's diet seems very important in establishing optimal choline levels for the developing fetus. Also, mother's milk, being higher in lecithin than cow's milk, may be extremely important in providing optimal levels of choline for the developing nervous system of the infant.[11]

## THERAPEUTIC BENEFITS OF CHOLINE/LECITHIN ADMINISTRATION

Choline has been used to treat certain neurological diseases for over fifty years. The major sites of action when choline is given therapeutically are the nervous system, the cardiovascular system and the liver. In the nervous system, choline has been found to stimulate the production of acetylcholine in the brain. Acetylcholine is used as a neurotransmitter involved in arousal learning, REM sleep and motor activity.[12]

Therapeutically, it has been used in doses of about 9 to 12 grams of choline chloride per day to treat tardive dyskinesia, a neurological condition produced as a side effect of the use of anti-schizophrenic medication. Tardive dyskinesia results when there is inadequate manufacture of acetylcholine in certain neurons in the brain. Enhanced levels of dietary choline or lecithin will normalize this synthesis and remove the symptoms of fine motor shaking, slurred speech and palsy-like reactions of the nervous system. All known neuroleptic drugs can produce tardive dyskinesia as a side effect. These conditions appear in approximately 50 percent of the patients treated with these medications. At this time the only effective treatment for tardive dyskinesia is the administration of therapeutic doses of oral choline or lecithin, with lecithin apparently preferable to choline.[13]

Other motor problems such as Huntington's disease and Gilles de la Tourette syndrome have also been suggested to be responsive to enhanced dietary choline or lecithin.

One of the clinical applications of enhanced lecithin and choline consumption is improved memory in the presenile demented patient. Memory loss in these patients seems to be a result of the loss of acetylcholine in the septohypocampal cholinergic neuron in the brain. Enhanced dietary levels of lecithin or choline will override this difficulty.[14] It is well known that even healthy humans who are treated with anticholinergic drugs may develop memory loss; the use of dietary supplements of lecithin or choline can reduce these symptoms.

Alzheimer's disease is a condition associated with memory loss in the aged individual and has been suggested to be related to excessive aluminum exposure and concentration of aluminum in the brain. Recently, lecithin has been found helpful in the Alzheimer's disease patient.

One exciting development in the use of lecithin therapeutically is in the management of manic depression or bipolar disorder along with lithium. Lithium improves the uptake of choline across the blood/brain barrier, and the administration of lecithin along with lithium will reduce the need for lithium considerably, thereby improving the levels of acetylcholine. Seventy-five percent of patients in a clinical trial when taken off choline enrichment but kept only on lithium worsened with regard to their manic depression.[15]

Lecithin seems preferable in these uses to that of choline. Choline must be administered four times a day at levels of 2½ to 3 grams per administration to keep the blood levels in the therapeutic range, whereas lecithin is like a time-released choline and only needs to be administrated twice daily.

It is important to point out, however, that the use of lecithin and success with it is dependent upon the quality of the lecithin as it relates to its phosphatidylcholine content. For therapeutic success to result, the lecithin must be at least 30 percent phosphatidylcholine, with the higher levels having even more clinical success.[16] Many commercially available lecithins do not have this degree of concentration of phosphatidylcholine and are heavily diluted with other oils, and therefore will not be clinically useful.

Lecithin has also been useful in increasing acetylcholine levels in the peripheral nervous system and may help in thyroid-and adrenal-related hypertension (or elevated blood pressure) problems.

## LECITHIN AND SERUM CHOLESTEROL

Early clinical trials have failed to confirm that lecithin is useful in improving HDL levels or reducing blood cholesterol.[17] However, it has since been shown that lecithin can keep cholesterol from damaging arteries. The emulsifying factors of lecithin help to make cholesterol more soluble and thus prevent cholesterol gallstones. Other dietary variables which influence the composition of bile include copper, vitamin B12, folic acid and the amino acid methionine, as well as vitamin C.

In conclusion, it can be seen that choline and lecithin (preferably lecithin) can be used therapeutically, particularly in certain neurological disorders characterized by insufficient acetylcholine synthesis in the neurons of the brain. These substances are also useful in the treatment of memory loss in the elderly, tardive dyskinesia and Alzheimer's disease-like symptoms, as well as peripheral nervous system improvement, particularly those connected to thyroid- and adrenal-related high blood pressure problems.

## DIETARY SOURCES OF INOSITOL

The accessory food factor inositol is found in plants as inositol phosphate, sometimes called phytate. This material serves as a source of phosphorus in the plant during the germination process. The germination of a seed or grain will cause phosphatase enzymes to chemically cleave the phosphate groups off phytate, liberating inositol.

Inositol can be manufactured within the human body as well as in plant products, but again, its level of manufacture in certain individuals may not be optimal for their health. The dietary requirement in humans is uncertain but it is known that the synthesis occurs in the liver and by bacteria in the intestinal tract. There have been deficiencies identified in some tissues, and these symptoms include irritability, insomnia, hyperexcitability and nervousness.[18]

Dietary sources of inositol generally occur as myo-inositol and seem to be essential for the survival and growth of every human cell type that has been examined to date. It is interesting that diets high in unsprouted seeds and grains, which are thereby rich in phytates, may prevent the proper absorption of many trace elements in the diet, since phytates very effectively bind, or chelate the minerals in the diet, rendering them less absorbable. Either leavening of the grains or germination prior to their use will eliminate the phytates, liberating only inositol into the final food product.

### PHYSIOLOGICAL FUNCTION OF INOSITOL

Inositol is another member of the lipotrophic vitamin family of nutrients which prevents fatty liver infiltration and works along with folic acid, vitamin B12, vitamin B6, choline and betaine, and the amino acid methionine in stimulating proper liver management of fats.[19]

Antibiotics which lead to sterilization of the intestine prevent inositol synthesis and may induce a deficiency symptom. Lactation without adequate inositol in the diet can cause reduction in body inositol stores and lead to fatty liver syndrome in the baby even if the mother is on a low-fat diet.

Clinically, it has been found that individuals on a low inositol diet have a reduction in high-density lipoprotein cholesterol (HDL) but not low-density lipoprotein cholesterol (LDL). The reduction in HDL levels may indicate increased risk of coronary heart disease; HDL appears to be a protective form of cholesterol to atherosclerotic disease.[20]

Inositol has been found to function as a cell growth factor, since it stimulates the manufacture in the body of complex phospholipids, or a class of fats used in the body for the manufacture of myelinated nerve material. Inappropriately low amounts of inositol can reduce nerve growth and regeneration.

The most important clinical manifestation of this observation is the recent work which has indicated that peripheral neurological complications of diabetes which involve pain in the hands and feet, tingling sensation, and numbness of the fingers and toes with reduced nerve conduction velocity can be treated by administering large therapeutic doses of inositol as a supplement.[21] This condition of peripheral neuritis is responsive to myo-inositol supplementation at levels of 1000 to 3000 mg per day. The average American 2500 kilocalorie diet contains 900 mg of inositol, with most specialists claiming that this amount is more than adequate to meet the daily needs. In diabetics with peripheral neuritis, however, the level of inositol in the average diet is not high enough to be in the effective therapy range. When there is an increase from 770 to 1640 mg per day of inositol, there is a significant improvement in the sensory neurons of diabetics with neuropathy. The level of 1600 mg can be achieved by careful selection of certain foods for the diet, but in general it is very difficult to achieve from dietary sources alone and an inositol supplement may be required.[22] Table 1 outlines the foods highest in inositol with the corresponding amounts given per 100 gram edible portion of the foods.

Salaway, in a clinical trial, used 1000 mg per day of inositol as a tablet in diabetics to increase action potentials of nerves and nerve conduction velocity and has successfully managed peripheral neuropathy in many diabetics using this method.[22]

## THERAPEUTIC USE OF INOSITOL

Inositol is one of those important therapeutic nutritional agents which will find significant application in the management of neuropathy, particularly associated with diabetes and the attendant pain that occurs as a result of demyelinating conditions of the nerves. This demyelinization is similar to an electrical wire losing its insulation and starting to short out. The stimulation of the synthesis of the proper nervous system material occurs with therapeutic doses of inositol between 1000 and 3000 mg of inositol per day, some of which may be derived from a diet higher in beans, oranges, cantaloupes, grapefruit or whole wheat, and the balance by way of a supplemental dose.

TABLE 1. MYO-INOSITOL CONTENT OF SELECTED FOODS[21]

| Food | Serving | mg/serving |
|---|---|---|
| Pole beans | ½ cup | 175 |
| Green beans, shelled | ½ cup | 193 |
| Cantaloupe | ¼ | 355 |
| Orange, fresh | 1 | 307 |
| Grapefruit, fresh | ½ | 199 |
| Lime | 1 | 194 |
| Grapefruit juice | ½ cup | 456 |
| Orange juice | ½ cup | 244 |
| Whole-wheat bread (stone ground) | 1 slice | 287 |
| Beans, cooked | ½ cup | 283 |

## THE FUTURE DIRECTION AND USEFULNESS OF THE ACCESSORY NUTRIENT FAMILY

In this short chapter we have explored the clinical utility of accessory food factors. This is just a small sampling of the total family of substances that are now known when concentrated from food to have clinical utility at therapeutic levels in specific individuals. It should be remembered that for one individual an accessory food factor may not be required because his or her body is capable of manufacturing adequate levels, whereas in another individual that factor may be an essential nutrient, either because of the metabolic inability to manufacture the substance or a specific disease process that may require augmented supplies to normalize function.

It is clear that not all individuals should be supplementing with accessory food factors, but that for those individuals who have specific metabolic or health requirements these agents when given therapeutically can prove extremely helpful in promoting health and proper function.

As we learn more about this exciting family of food concentrates and their implications on improving cellular function in specific individuals, the list of these agents will grow and become better established. The future is bright for this area of clinical nutrition but is one that will be continuously fraught with controversy, because these substances do not have a distinct deficiency symptom associated with their absence in the diet, but rather long-term evidence that their absence in adequate amounts may lead to chronic impairment of health. Most of our understanding of the essential nutrients is built around the concept that absence from the diet produces a deficiency disease, as the absence of vitamin C leading to scurvy and the absence of the B-complex vitamins leading to beri-beri or pellagra.

In the case of the accessory food factors, however, there is no acute deficiency disease which results from their absence because the body is able to manufacture some by its own processes. The challenge before the clinical nutritionist who is exploring the role and usefulness of members of the accessory food factor family is to identify those people who are at risk to deficiency of these agents and who have inherent need for supplementation of one or more of this family. We are now in the process of addressing these problems and more clearly defining where these substances have clinical utility.

## REFERENCES

1. Fujimoto, A. and Bessman, S. P. 1978. *American Journal of Human Genetics* 30:51A.
2. Bessman, S. P. 1978. *Nutrition Reviews* 37:209-220.
3. Williams, R. J. and Deason, G. 1968. *Proceedings National Academy of Sciences* 57:1638-1642.
4. Horrobin, D. F. and Manku, M. S. 1980. *British Medical Journal* 280:1363-1366.
5. Culp, B. R., Lands, W. E. M. and Romson, J. 1980. *Prostaglandins* 20:1021-1031.
6. Zeisel, S. H. 1981. *Annual Reviews of Nutrition* 1:95-115.
7. Beams, A. J. 1946. *Journal American Medical Association* 130:190-196.
8. Zeisel, S. H., Growdon, J. H. and Wurtman, R. J., 1980. *Proceedings of National Academy of Sciences* 77:4417-4419.
9. Kapp, J., Mahaley, M. S. and Odom, G. L. 1970. *J. Neurosurgery* 32:468-472.
10. Rama Sastry, B. V. and Schmidt, D. E. 1976. *Biochemistry and Pharmacology* 25:425-431.
11. Jensen, R. G., Hagerty, M. M. and McMahon, K. E. 1978. *American Journal of Clinical Nutrition* 31:990-1016.
12. McGeer, P. L. and McGeer, E. G. 1979. *Nutrition and the Brain.* New York: Raven Press, pp. 141-176.
13. Davis, K. L., Berger, P. A. and Hollister, L. E. 1975. *New England Journal of Medicine* 293:152.
14. Boyd, W. D. and McQueen, J. 1977. *Lancet* 2:711.
15. Cohen, B. M., Miller, A. L. and Lipinski, J. 1980. *American Journal of Psychiatry* 137:242-243.
16. Steigmann, F., Finestein, R. and De La Huerga, J. 1952. *Federation Proceedings* 11:393.

17. Ter Well, H. F., Van Gent, C. M. and Dekker, W. 1974. *Acta Med. Scandinavian* 195:267-271.
18. Kuksis, A. and MooKerjea, S. 1978. *Nutrition Reviews* 36:233-237.
19. Gavin, G. and McHenry, E. W. 1941. *Journal Biological Chemistry* 139:485.
20. Ockner, R. K., Hughes, F. B. and Isselbacher, K. J. 1969. *Journal Clinical Investigation* 48:2367-2371.
21. Clements, R. S. and Darnell, B. 1980. *American Journal Clinical Nutrition* 33:1954-1967.
22. Salaway, J. G., Whitehead, L. and Payne, R. E. 1978. *Lancet* December 16, pp. 1282-1284.

# OCTACOSANOL, CARNITINE AND TAURINE

## *Make the Most of Your Health With Nutrients Your Own Body Needs*

**JEFFREY BLAND, PH.D.**

Accessory food factors are nutrients that may be manufactured within the human body and therefore are not considered essential nutrients as such. (The term "essential" means that the substance is not manufactured within the human body, but is necessary for survival and so must be gotten from the diet.) The use of these accessory factors such as carnitine and taurine, both of which are manufactured within the body, is for specific therapeutic need in the individuals who are incapable of manufacturing the amount necessary for optimal health. Concentration of these principles from natural food sources can then lead to the formulation of specific food supplements for individuals who require more of the specific agent than they can manufacture. This can be called nutritional pharmacology, a new branch of clinical nutrition that recognizes the function of certain food concentrates in the management of specific individuals.[1]

A review article by Bessman[2] has pointed out that even amino acids generally considered "nonessential" for most individuals may be essential for a few people who do not have adequate ability to manufacture them within their own bodies. Bessman calls this the justification theory that indicates, on the basis of an individual's unique genetic nature when a nonessential nutrient may become an essential nutrient. The use of this accessory food factor in supplemental doses becomes "essential" for that individual's good health.

Three such examples of these therapeutic nutrients are octacosanol, carnitine and taurine. None of these substances will be found listed in the tables of essential nutrients for humans; however, each has found specific therapeutic value in certain individuals. It should be remembered that *nutrition is for real individuals.* The statistical human or the average man is of little value in assessing the need for therapeutic nutrition.

Historically, the nutritionists' interest has been the study of the effects of essential nutrients in food on the biochemical and physiological function of humans. In this volume, this interest has been expanded to include accessory substances within foods which may be used therapeutically to help specific individuals with a pharmacological need.[3]

## OCTACOSANOL

For millennia, early humans ate diets high in unrefined grains which were rich in unsaturated oils, vegetable fats and waxes. As our diets grew more processed and refined, many of these oils in their natural state were removed. As a result of these dietary changes, animal fat began to replace the natural oils and fat principles found in whole wheat, rye, corn and millet. Wheat germ was one of the foods highest in unsaturated oil content, as well as a rich source of vitamin E and protein. In the 1930s a commercial process to extract the oils from wheat germ was developed and when these oils were administered in the diets of human volunteers, improvement in endurance and stamina was observed. Studies by William Smiley[4] and Charles White[5] in the 1950s indicated reduced oxygen stress and quickened reaction time in exercise studies done on trained and untrained individuals. Later Ershoff and Levin found a beneficial effect of an unidentified factor in wheat germ oil on the swimming performance of guinea pigs.[6] This observation set the biochemists to work to determine what the principle or principles in wheat germ oil might be that helped improve exercise tolerance. At first it was thought that it might be vitamin E, but later it was concluded that the observed beneficial effects were not due to vitamin E. Studies on animals confirmed that there was a significant difference in the therapeutic benefit of vitamin E and wheat germ oil, with the wheat germ oil principle being superior for improving endurance.[7]

The chemical principles of wheat germ oil were finally established to include essential fatty acids such as linoleic acid, vitamin E, and a high boiling residue made up of long-chain alcohols and plant sterols. The long-chain alcohols included octacosanol, triacontanol, tetracosanol and hexacosanol. A commercial process was developed and patented by Ezra Levin to extract these long-chain alcohols from wheat germ oil, and human studies were started by Dr. Thomas Cureton on the effect of these substances on improving stamina and exercise tolerance. The patent held by Levin (patented April 24, 1962, No. 3,031,376) led to the production of a wheat germ oil concentrate high in several long-chain alcohols and neutral plant sterols.

## CLINICAL UTILITY

Studies by Alfin-Slater indicated that this unidentified complex mixture of substances was capable of decreasing blood cholesterol.[8] Work by Vahouny and Kritchevsky[9] indicated that this was a result of the high plant sterol content of beta-sitosterol in wheat germ oil which blocks excessive blood cholesterol.

Cureton found that factors in this wheat germ oil concentrate which improved endurance seemed to be related to octacosanol, the 28 carbon straight chain, saturated alcohol.[10] Work by Farrell in animals confirmed that these long-chain alcohols improved oxygen utilization.[11]

The studies on humans who were administered doses of this concentrate orally, equivalent to 1000 micrograms of octacosanol and

2000 micrograms of the other naturally occurring long-chain alcohols, indicated:

1. Improved muscle glycogen storage
2. Stability of basal metabolic rate under stress
3. Reduced high altitude stress
4. Improved reaction time
5. Reduced oxygen debt
6. Improved endurance.

## COMMERCIAL PROCESS

These clinical studies were all done with the natural concentrate from wheat germ oil, manufactured by the Levin process (Viobin Corporation). Recently, purified octacosanol has become available from nonwheat-germ sources. These products make label claim of very high octacosanol content, but it should be pointed out that these are not the products used by Cureton in his clinical studies. The usefulness of the wheat germ oil concentrate may very well be due to its complex synergistic mixture of various alcohols and plant sterols. Highly purified, petrochemically originated octacosanol cannot offer this complex mixture of natural materials. The burden of proof for clinical usefulness of these pure octacosanol products is on the shoulders of the manufacturers. Failure to achieve the desired results with octacosanol concentrates may be due to the product quality and composition. The naturally derived wheat germ oil concentrate remains the only clinically proven substance that has ergogenic activity (improvement of oxygen utilization when exercising).

It is possible to get these principles from whole grains, but it should be pointed out that ten pounds of whole wheat are concentrated to give 1000 micrograms equivalent of octacosanol under the Levin process.

In sum, the therapeutic use of wheat germ oil concentrate has support in clinical studies for improved exercise tolerance, reduced blood cholesterol, improved oxygen utilization, and as a neuromuscular factor to prohibit muscle pain after exercise.[12] Muscular dystrophies and other neuromuscular disorders have proven responsive to wheat germ oil concentrate.[13] The wheat germ oil concentrate used in Dr. Thomas Cureton's studies which indicated the positive effect of this substance on exercise and oxygen utilization can be considered the application of therapeutic nutrition. It is not a supplement required necessarily by everyone, but its effect in improving oxygen utilization and in lowering blood cholesterol may be most helpful for those individuals who experience muscle pain after exercise, poor exercise tolerance or lowered endurance.

## CARNITINE

### DIETARY SOURCES AND FUNCTION

Carnitine is an unusual amino acid that is biosynthesized in the liver of humans and is found highest in muscle and organ meats in the human diet. Carnitine is not found in vegetable sources. In human metabolism it is utilized as a material which transfers fatty acids across the membranes of the mitochondria (which are like the lungs of the cell) where they can be used as a source of fuel to generate energy. In the absence of proper carnitine levels within the cell, the fatty acids are poorly metabolized and can build up within the cell or the surrounding medium, thereby leading to elevated blood fat and triglyceride levels.[14]

Carnitine has been found to have an important regulatory effect upon fat metabolism in heart and skeletal muscles. The administration of carnitine in tissue culture has been shown to stimulate fat metabolism and encourage the clearance of triglycerides and fatty acids.[15]

Carnitine is not a vitamin, because it can be manufactured in the human body, but it is somewhat like the relationship of niacin to tryptophan[16] It is well known that niacin can be partially manufactured from tryptophan, but not in adequate amounts to prevent a niacin deficiency, called pellagra. Carnitine likewise is manufactured in the body from the amino acids lysine and methionine, but again not at levels adequate to meet the needs of all individuals, particularly if they are on a low lysine or methionine diet. It should be pointed out that lysine and methionine are both essential amino acids found in adequate levels in high quality protein, but which may be deficient in unbalanced vegetable protein. The reliance upon a single vegetable protein family such as wheat, soy or corn could lead to specific deficiencies of lysine or methionine and could contribute to an imbalance in the manufacture of carnitine. This may explain why some vegetarians who are on poorly balanced vegetarian diets have elevated blood fats, such as triglycerides, because of carnitine insufficiency.

There has also been found a considerable difference in the level of need for carnitine between men and women. Men have higher blood carnitine than women, and high levels of carnitine are found in the epididymis of the testes in men.[17] The spermatozoa from lysine-depleted animals became infertile due to potential carnitine insufficiency. This is the first tissue to show deficiencies in animals that have been deprived of carnitine or lysine. Adequate levels of carnitine are necessary for energy metabolism within the sperm for proper motility and fertility[18]

The synthesis of carnitine from lysine and methionine necessitates vitamin C. The role of vitamin C in the manufacture of carnitine is similar to the role that vitamin C plays in the manufacture of hydroxyproline, an amino acid used in the manufacture of collagen, a connective tissue. Working with vitamin C in the manufacture of carnitine are vitamin B6, niacin, lysine and methionine. Low levels of vitamin C intake have also been indicated to produce symptoms of carnitine deficiency, and this is why scurvy may be associated with a high level of blood fat.[19]

Although carnitine has not been recognized as a vitamin, it may be required by newborns as a vitamin, because their bio-synthetic machinery is late to develop and may be unavailable for proper carnitine biosynthesis. There seem to be genetic limitations on the ability of some individuals to synthesize carnitine from lysine or methionine, and therefore in these individuals carnitine may be an essential nutrient.[20]

## CLINICAL REPORTS OF DEFICIENCY

Engel and Angelini reported the first carnitine deficiency in humans in 1972.[21] In this case, they report infiltration of the liver with fat and depressed muscle carnitine levels with generalized spleen and liver enlargement and muscle wasting. Human carnitine deficiencies, which have been identified since 1972, range from actual deficiencies of carnitine due to dietary and biosynthetic unavailability to transport problems of carnitine as it relates to the inability of individuals to transport carnitine in their blood to the cells of need.

Chapoy and coworkers recognized a carnitine deficiency which resembled Reye syndrome.[22] The case history was that of a 6-month-old boy who had heart failure, an enlarged liver, gross retardation, infections of the respiratory tract, with fatty liver and low liver carnitine levels. After a number of years of not knowing what was wrong with the boy it was finally recognized that he might be suffering from a carnitine deficiency. He was then given 4000 mg per day of carnitine and showed remarkable improvement almost immediately. Over a period of two years his health changed for the better and it was determined that he was suffering from a defect in the enzyme responsible for the manufacture of carnitine from lysine and methionine. The effective treatment of this youngster led to the mobilization of fat from the heart and muscle, a diminution of the heart size, improved muscle strength and improved neurological function.

## THERAPEUTIC USE OF CARNITINE

The most exciting recent advances in the use of carnitine in clinical nutrition is as an agent to improve fat metabolism and to reduce blood triglycerides when 1000 to 3000 mg of dl-carnitine are administered daily.[23] Elevated triglycerides can lead to increased risk to small vessel diseases, such as poor circulation in the hands and feet, kidney problems and the inability to walk without pain, called claudication. The management of this problem by utilizing a lower fat diet with lower sugar and increased carnitine as a supplement has effectively reduced triglycerides in patients who have blood triglyceride levels of 800 to 1000 mg/100 ml (normal range less than 150 mg/100 ml).

Neuromuscular diseases such as certain myopathies or problems with the heart, muscular dystrophy, myotonic dystrophy and limb-girdle muscular dystrophy have all been suggested to be aided or improved by administration of carnitine as a supplement. There is some indication that these neuromuscular diseases lead to an increased loss of carnitine in the urine and therefore may require higher levels for adequacy.[24]

Carnitine has also been found to be helpful in those people who want to improve fatty acid metabolism due to metabolic obesity problems. Many weight-loss diets cause a problem called ketosis which is the accumulation of ketone bodies or fat waste products in the blood.

### CARNITINE AND MALE INFERTILITY

The lower the concentration of the amino acid L-carnitine in male sperm, the lower the sperm count and motility and the more likely the man is to be infertile. A recent study reported in *Andrologia* (26:1994) assessed the therapeutic effect of a four-month trial of 3,000 mg of carnitine a day in 100 infertile men with low sperm counts. The results of the study showed an increase in both sperm count and sperm motility, with the most dramatic gains in those patients who entered the study with the poorest sperm motility.

These ketones can cause the blood to become acid and lead to the loss of calcium, magnesium and potassium in the urine. Ketosis when uncontrolled in poor weight-loss diets or diabetes can be life-threatening. The use of carnitine in therapeutic doses as a food supplement can encourage the proper metabolism of fats and prevent ketones from building up in people who are susceptible to ketosis.[25] Prevention of ketosis can be the difference between a poorly controlled and well-controlled weight-loss diet.

The future of this accessory food factor in clinical nutrition is very rich, and as studies are made to indicate specifically the various forms of neuromuscular and fatty acid diseases that may respond to supplements of carnitine, its application in health care will increase.

## TAURINE

### DIETARY SOURCES AND FUNCTION

Taurine is another amino acid which is manufactured in the human body and therefore is not considered an essential nutrient. It is known to be a neurotransmitter in the central nervous system of humans and other animals, but it has only been identified as an essential nutrient in cats. Taurine is found only in animal products and not in vegetable protein sources. It is a sulfur amino acid derivative, and this may indicate why cats on soy protein diets or heavy vegetable-based protein diets may develop certain types of neurological and behavioral changes.[26]

Taurine was first derived from ox bile, where it is found in high concentration. In the human it is biosynthesized from the amino acids cysteine and methionine, which are two sulfur amino acids found in high quality dietary protein. Vegetarians who are on imbalanced dietary proteins of lower quality may have difficulty manufacturing adequate levels of taurine.

Most taurine in humans is synthesized in the liver, and there is only a limited ability for this synthesis. Vitamin B6 has been found necessary for the manufacture of taurine in the liver from methionine and cysteine.

Women may have much more need for taurine in the diet than men since the female hormone estradiol is found to inhibit the synthesis of taurine in the liver. Certain estrogenic hormone substances when given to women may therefore increase the inhibition of taurine synthesis and require even more dietary intake.[27]

Taurine is found in the brain as a neurotransmitter working along with the other neuroinhibitory transmitters gamma aminobutyric acid (GABA) and glycine. Large oral doses of taurine have been found to increase growth hormone in animals.

Taurine also conjugates chemically with bile acids in the liver. This seems to be very important for the maintenance of proper bile composition and for keeping cholesterol soluble. The liver is the only tissue where taurine has metabolized, although there have been high levels found in the retina, brain and heart.[28]

Taurine works by itself as a single amino acid substance and it has been found to be concentrated in the pineal and pituitary glands in higher levels when the individual has been exposed to full spectrum light.[29] A deficiency of exposure to the near ultraviolet portion of the spectrum (which occurs when an individual is only exposed to fluorescent lights or incandescent bulbs) may lead to impaired concentration of the neurotransmitter taurine in the pineal and pituitary glands.

Increased urinary spill of taurine has been found when individuals have been placed under stress. Taurine works with zinc in the eyes, and deficiencies of taurine have led to functional impairment of vision well before there was an actual structural alteration of the eye.[30] In animals, depletion of taurine occurs slowly, but eventually leads to blindness. Between 25 and 90 percent of the taurine in the body is conjugated to bile salts, and this makes the bile less lithogenic or prevents cholesterol gallstones.

Taurine is the second most abundant amino acid in human milk, and infants may need taurine above what is found in cow's milk or a soy formula. Being without it may lead to growth depression, as has been shown in many primates such as monkeys and apes.[31]

## NEUROLOGICAL DISORDERS AND TAURINE

Taurine's role in the central nervous system is that of an inhibitory neurotransmitter. Deficiencies of taurine may produce memory loss, although the results are not very reproducible in this area. The brain is in subtle balance between the messages coming from the neuroexcitatory transmitters, such as the serotonin and dopamine family, and the neuroinhibitory transmitters, such as GABA and taurine. When there is a deficiency of the neuroinhibitory transmitters, there is an over-excitation of certain portions of the brain which may lead to convulsions. Because of this observation, Huxtable and Barbeau attempted to use oral doses of taurine in the treatment of epilepsy or as an anticonvulsant in drug toxicities.[32] They found that taurine influenced the movement of calcium ions in the brain, and that the observed anticonvulsant effects of taurine may be a result of this biochemical effect. Taurine undoubtedly serves both as a neurotransmitter and a neuromodulator substance in the management of central nervous system function.

## POTASSIUM-SPARING EFFECTS OF TAURINE

An additional important role that taurine plays is to spare the loss of potassium from the heart muscle. Recent evidence indicates that taurine may be the critical substance in the osmotic regulation of both calcium and potassium concentrations within the heart muscle and in preventing potassium or calcium wasting, particularly during times of weight-loss dieting.[33] It is well known that the heart irregularities in a number of people who were on the liquid protein diets a few years back were very similar to those produced during times of potassium depletion. This seemed unusual, since many of the people on these diets were actually on potassium supplementation. Follow-up studies indicated that many of the liquid protein weight-loss products were low in the amino acids cysteine or methionine, and thereby may have led to the inability of the heart muscle to retain potassium and to the observed heart problems.[34] It can be seen then that proper amounts of taurine seem essential to prevent potassium and calcium loss from the heart during biochemical stress on a weight-loss diet. Those proteins which are rich in the sulfur amino acids should especially be supplied at those times to avoid taurine deficiency.

## TAURINE AND NUTRITIONAL INDIVIDUALITY

Taurine has also been found to resemble the effect of insulin on blood sugar. It seems to promote the proper regulation of blood sugar in the individual who may be insulin insufficient.[35]

Vitamin A and vitamin E deficiency lead to increased taurine excretion with greater need for intake. Recently these vitamins have been found to play some role in the management of muscular dystrophy, although this work is still in the early stages of clinical investigation.[36]

The whole array of metabolic genetic problems associated with sulfur amino acid metabolism, of which many are known, may indicate a dietary increased need for taurine. Conditions such as homocystinuria or cystathioninuria, which are known to be vitamin B6 dependent, may also indicate the need for supplemental taurine.

Lastly, taurine has been intimated to be a limiting nutrient in some forms of mental retardation, such as in Down syndrome. Studies are now under way to look at the effect on intelligence quotient in those Down syndrome children who are supplemented with taurine. This accessory food factor may work along with the B-complex vitamins and vitamins C and E in the improvement of intelligence in mentally retarded individuals.[37]

Taurine is one of those remarkable accessory food factors whose therapeutic use is just now beginning to be understood. Its panoramic effects cover functional applications from the management of some forms of epilepsy to the prevention of potassium and calcium loss from the heart muscle to improved bile composition and the prevention of gallstones. It should be recalled that dietary taurine comes exclusively from animal products, and is related to the sulfur amino acids; therefore, metabolic defects in the metabolism of the sulfur amino acids may lead to insufficiencies of taurine and require augmented dietary intake.

## SUMMARY

The accessory food factors we have discussed are representative of the explosion of information that is occurring in this branch of therapeutic nutrition. As more and more principles from various foods are concentrated and shown to have clinical response in certain individuals with needs determined by their own individual biochemistry, this field of therapeutic nutrition will grow ever more important.

All in all, these accessory food factors frame a class of substances that may prove vital for certain individuals in making the most of their health and wellness and serving as a useful adjunct to an improved diet. The thrust of the research indicates clearly that what is optimal nutrition for one may not be for another and that essential nutrients may be different from individual to individual, based upon the needs of each one. Octacosanol, carnitine and taurine are three representative examples of these substances which may prove some degree of "essentiality" for optimal health in a specific individual. This field of therapeutic nutrition will continue to explode with major health improvement resulting from this research.

## REFERENCES


1. Spiller, G. A. 1982. Nutritional Pharmacology volume 4, in *Current Topics in Nutrition and Disease.* New York: Alan Liss, Inc.
2. Bessman, S. P. 1979. *Nutrition Reviews* 37, 209-211.
3. Spiller, G. A. 1980. *American Journal of Clinical Nutrition* 33, 1716-1719.
4. Smiley, W. A. 1951. Variations on a bicycle ergometer test with altitude, training, and a dietary supplement. M.S. thesis. University of Illinois.

5. White, C. H. 1951. The effect of physical training and a dietary supplement on the six Schneider index tests. M.S. thesis. University of Illinois.
6. Ershoff, B. A., and Levin, E. 1955. *Federation Proceedings* 14, 431-437.
7. Dukelow, W. R. 1963. *Acta Endocrinologica* pp. 5-15.
8. Alfin-Slater, R. B. 1960. *Federation Proceedings* 19, 18-22.
9. Deuel, H. J. 1951. *The Lipids.* New York: Wiley-Interscience p. 361; also see reference 1, pp. 31-72.
10. Cureton, T. K. 1958. *Med. Sportiva* 12, 259-263.
11. Farrell, P. R. 1965. Effects of octacosanol on conception and oxygen uptake in the white rat. M.S. thesis. Kansas State University.
12. Bicknell, F. 1940. *The Lancet,* pp. 10-11.
13. Stone, S. 1941. *Journal of American Medical Association* 18, 310-312.
14. Bremer, J. 1977. *Trends in Biochemical Sciences* 2, 207-209.
15. McGarry, J. D. and Foster, D. W. 1975. *Proceedings National Academy Sciences* 72, 4385-4388.
16. Broquist, H. P. 1976. *Nutrition Reviews* 34, 289-293.
17. Cederblad, G. 1977. *Clinical Chem. Acta* 67, 207-212.
18. Borum, P. R. and Broquist, H. P. 1977. *Journal Nutrition* 107, 1209-1215.
19. Hulse, J. D., Ellis, S. R. and Henderson, L. M. 1978. *Journal of Biological Chemistry* 253, 1654-1659.
20. Borum, P. 1981. *Nutrition Reviews* 39, 385-390.
21. Engel, A. G. and Angelini, C. 1973. *Science* 179, 899-902.
22. Chapoy, P. R., Angelini, C. and Brown, W. J. 1980. *New England Journal of Medicine* 303, 1389-1394.
23. Maebashi, M; Sato, M.; Immura, A.; and Yoshinaga, K. 1978. *Lancet,* October 14.
24. Carroll, J. E.; Brooke, M. H.; Shumate, J. B.; and Janes, N. J. 1981. *American Journal of Clinical Nutrition* 34, 2693-2698.
25. Mitchell, M. E. 1978. *American Journal of Clinical Nutrition* 31, 645-659.
26. Hayes, K.C. and Sturman, J. A. 1981. *Annual Reviews of Nutrition 1,* 401-425.
27. Awapara, J. 1976. In *Taurine,* ed., R. Huxtable, A. Barbeau pp. 1-19.
28. Baskin, S. I. and Finney, C. M. 1979. *Sulfur-Amino Acids 2,* 1-18.
29. Grosso, D. S., Bressler, R. and Benson, B. 1978. *Life-Sciences 22,* 1789-1798.
30. McLardy, T. 1962. *Nature* 194, 300-302.

31. Gaull, G. E., Rassia, D. K. and Heinonen, K. 1977. *Journal Pediatrics* 90, 348-355.
32. Barbeau, A. and Butterworth, R. F. 1975. *Life Sciences* 17, 669-677.
33. Thurston, J. H., Hauhart, R. E. and Naccarato, E. F. 1981. *Science* 214, 1373-1374.
34. Feldman, J. 1980. *Obesity and Bariatric Medicine* 9, 12-16.
35. McCallum, A. B. and Divertz, C. 1942. *Canadian Chemical Process Industry* 26, 569-570.
36. Gruener, R. and Huxtable, R. 1975. *Journal of Neurological Sciences* 24, 351-360.
37. Harrell, R. F., Capp, R. H. and Davis, D. R. 1981. *Proceedings National Academy of Sciences* 78, 574-578.

# SESAME

## *The Superfood Seed and How It Can Add Vitality to Your Life*

BETTY KAMEN, PH.D.

THE GOURMET NUTRIENT

Sesame seeds, with their unusual amino acid profile, complement many other foods to build complete protein, adding nourishment and unique flavor to main dishes, dips, dressings, baked goods, desserts and refreshing drinks. Learn why sesame is such a powerhouse of health benefits, and how to use it for more enjoyable, more healthy eating.

## INTRODUCTION

They say there is nothing new under the sun. Indeed there isn't, and this even applies to the information in this chapter. For thousands of years healthful seeds and grains have been combined to produce meals of complete protein, a process called "protein complementarity." Imagine such wisdom without benefit of any knowledge of amino acids (the component parts of protein). In the long climb to the world we now know, the practice of successful protein combining was lost until recently, but only in modern countries such as ours.

Information on protein and vegetarianism fill the pages of current accepted medical literature. Journals and technical books include the results of experience and studies for and by professionals from around the world. But it takes many years for the conclusions to filter through, and so this important subject remains unexplored in most late twentieth-century medical offices, kitchens and cookbooks in the United States.

The sesame seed is a crucial vehicle for defining protein complementarity concepts for several reasons. Sesame seeds contain:

- A unique amino acid profile, increasing protein value when combined with other foods
- A built-in resistance to rancidity, a problem common to other oil-bearing seeds
- A high natural polyunsaturated fat content, a substance almost totally lacking in the average American diet (yet optimal health depends on it!).

More than an exploration of the sesame seed, this chapter provides a valuable lesson in nutrition, demonstrating simple techniques for optimizing good quality, enhancing flavor, and even reducing the food budget. For example, you should know that there is a greater difference in protein quality between eggs and meat than there is between meat and vegetables. When you understand the value of sesame plus protein complementarity, this knowledge can be used to advantage.

## WHAT'S SO SPECIAL?

Thousands of food products line the shelves of your local supermarket. Many products result from recently acquired technological knowledge—foods are now available in forms that have been invented only recently. Why, then, should we even consider the nutritional value of a food such as sesame, which is both centuries old and unfamiliar to most of us (except for occasional recognition on a seeded roll)? Does it matter that the armies of Rome were known to have had sesame seed cakes as an energy ration? Does it matter that the very tough Turk and Greek soldiers carried sesame seeds at all times, right onto the battlefields? Does it matter that these seeds had a noble and illustrious past? Is sesame anything more than a flavor-enhancing condiment? This is, after all, the late twentieth century.

The answer to these questions is a simple statement of fact: Sesame seeds can enhance your health.

Known since at least the second century B.C., the sesame plant is believed to be indigenous to central Africa, and is now grown abundantly in Egypt. The production of olives in Egypt far from covers the country's oil needs, so sesame oil is used extensively, especially when animal fat cannot be used (either because of cost or religious prohibition). It is also a primary source of cooking oil in Africa and Asia, and it remains a staple item of the Iraqi diet.

Sesame was introduced to America by slaves who brought the seeds from Africa and cultivated them in the South, where it was used as a thickener and to lend flavor to special ethnic African foods. Today it serves mostly as a condiment in our country and in Europe.

Sesame is a hardy annual, partial to tropical climates, but it can be grown in temperate zones.

## NUTRITIONAL VALUE OF SESAME

Any seed will sprout when planted and watered, and, under proper growing conditions, become a new plant. The new plant proceeds to leaf out, flower and produce more seeds. Despite its size (one ounce contains thousands of seeds), sesame, like any other seed, has enough energy stored in it to rapidly become new life and to grow abundantly. Obviously, vitamins and minerals must be stored in the seed, waiting to participate in this energetic process. The nutrients in the seed must not only nourish the small plant while it matures, but they must also provide that spark which enables the seed to germinate, even after a long period of dormancy. Seeds represent the living force that carries one generation of plants to the next. That's why they're so healthful.

Most foods do not contain the full range of the nutrients required for health. If the nutritional profile of sesame seeds included vitamin

C and vitamin A, it would be an example of a perfect food that could be used as the sole item of diet because it possesses almost everything else that is nourishing.

## PROTEIN AND THE SESAME SEED

**Complementarity.** Suppose you have a bowl of alphabet soup and you need to pick out letters to assemble the entire alphabet. You will be able to create one complete set if you have each of the twenty-six letters. You could produce several sets if you have enough additional letters to go around. But if you are missing *one* letter, you are prevented from making even one complete set. So it is with protein. When you eat protein, your body takes that protein apart, separating the amino acids (the individual components of all protein). Then your body reassembles the amino acids into the unique pattern and sequence of human protein. It can only do this when it has the right amount of each amino acid that it needs to accomplish this function. Just as with the alphabet soup if you are in short supply of one amino acid, the other amino acids are useless.

Unused proteins are metabolized into urea, which concentrates in the blood and is filtered out by the kidneys. High levels of urea in the blood stream are reported to contribute to many serious problems, including fatigue.

The protein content of foods must be judged not only for quantity, but also for quality. Quality protein foods contain ratios of amino acids as close as possible to the ratio required for the human reassembly job. All foods contain all amino acids (even an apple contains all the amino acids), but protein that lacks quality usually lacks the necessary *quantity* of one or more amino acids necessary for the manufacture and repair of human tissue. We are just beginning to understand why it is that *quality* protein in your diet improves overall health.

The amino acids required can come from one food or several foods—your body doesn't really care where they come from, as long as they are all present and accounted for at the same time. Animal protein contains better ratios of amino acids, but such foods are usually accompanied by too much fat and/or other very objectionable substances that are not in your best health interest.

The strict vegetarian can increase protein value by using several techniques, among them:

1. consuming legumes—peas, beans, and lentils—in which the concentration of protein is high;
2. combining foods so that the weaknesses of one food (the limiting amino acids) are strengthened by the support of another (complementarity);
3. adding small amounts of animal protein to vegetable or grain dishes to boost protein quality.

As cited, complementarity is practiced worldwide. The best complementarity trick we know is that of adding mechanically hulled chemical-free sesame to grain and vegetable dishes, soups and salads. Sesame seeds provide two very important amino acids. One is methionine, which is in short supply in most vegetable foods and is crucial for maintaining healthy liver function. Sesame is one of the highest natural sources of methionine.

Every cell in your body requires methionine. When your body has its saturation of methionine, the excess is converted to choline—a nutrient usually on the deficiency list. Choline aids in the ability to handle cholesterol and helps the process by which the body produces energy instead of fat.

The second amino acid is tryptophan, reported to promote youthful skin and healthy hair, and known as the "tranquilizing nutrient." (Because turkey is high in tryptophan, it has been theorized that this is the reason everyone is ready for a nap after Thanksgiving dinner.)

Tryptophan is a precursor of niacin, thereby taking on the responsibility for a good nervous system since niacin helps maintain the health of blood vessels in the system.

Specific foods deficient in these two amino acids are peas, peanuts, wheat germ, soy, cottonseed, buckwheat flour and all beans including pinto, lima, mung and kidney.

**Comparative values.** A quarter of a pound of sesame seeds contains almost 19 grams of protein, which is as much protein as you would find in many meals. Let's compare the protein value of 100 grams of sesame seeds with several other food products. (Measurements of food products are usually stated in terms of 100 grams. An average portion or a fistful of food is about 100 grams.)

| Food | Protein Content |
|---|---|
| sesame seeds | 18.6% |
| navy beans | 7.8 |
| oatmeal | 14.2 |
| raw peas | 6.3 |
| rice polish | 12.1 |
| soybeans | 11.0 |
| lentils | 7.8 |
| eggs | 13.8 |

If you are not using sesame for protein balance, you may have to consume 50 percent more calories in a less efficient protein blend.

## SESAME AND B-COMPLEX

A quarter of a pound of sesame seeds contains a large percentage of the required B vitamins. Here are a few B-complex food comparisons.

| | Food | Milligrams per 100 Grams |
|---|---|---|
| Thiamin: | sesame seeds | .98 |
| | almonds | .24 |
| | navy beans | .14 |
| | mung beans | .38 |
| | lentils | .37 |
| | oatmeal | .34 |
| Riboflavin: | sesame seeds | .24 |
| | navy beans | .70 |
| | lentils | .22 |

| | Food | Milligrams per 100 Grams |
|---|---|---|
| | oatmeal | .14 |
| | peanuts | .13 |
| | raw peas | .14 |
| | rice polish | .18 |
| Niacin: | sesame seeds | 5.4 |
| | almonds | 3.5 |
| | navy beans | 0.7 |
| | mung beans | 2.6 |
| | cowpeas | 1.6 |
| | oatmeal | 1.0 |
| | raw peas | 2.9 |
| | soybeans | 2.2 |

## SESAME AND CARBOHYDRATES

A quarter of a pound of sesame seeds contains very little carbohydrate—only 21 grams. Note the comparative values.

| | Percent of carbohydrates 100 Grams |
|---|---|
| sesame seeds | 21.6% |
| mung beans | 60.3 |
| lentils | 60.1 |
| oatmeal | 68.2 |
| rice polish | 57.7 |
| soybeans | 33.5 |
| wheat germ | 46.7 |

## SESAME AND POLYUNSATURATED FATTY ACIDS

The seeds consist of about 55 percent oil, so that same quarter of a pound of sesame seeds contains about 49 grams of the finest unsaturated fat. Sesame seeds are called the "queen of the oilseed crops" because of the high quality of the seed, the meal and the oil.

The number one problem as viewed by the dermatologist is dry skin. According to very prestigious medical studies, essential fatty acid deficiency is usually the cause of dry skin.

Who has dry skin? More than half the people in this country. You probably have dry skin if your face feels like it's going to crack when you wash it; if you're more inclined to get whiteheads than blackheads; if your skin flakes, especially around the eyes, forehead, and nose; if your eye shadow and face powder don't go on smoothly; if your rouge is blotchy; and if you think you have more lines than a lot of other people your age. Dry skin may be the reason for itchiness, stretch marks, loosening dandruff, scaliness and flakiness on any part of your body. If you're not one to pay much attention to such details, you know you are a candidate for dry skin if you live in a cold, dry or windy climate, or one where there are extreme temperature changes from summer to winter. Recycled dry air (as in air conditioning) and exposure to noxious industrial and other air pollutants (as in living in a big city) may also be culprits. Even newborn infants may be affected. Babies often show biochemical signs of fatty acid deprivation as early as one week, and dermatitis may develop after three weeks. According to Dr. Irwin Lubowe, clinical professor of dermatology at New York Medical College, dry skin is the most common complexion problem among people of all ages in America.

But not everyone confronted with skin-drying promoters has dry skin. Your body should be able to transform the fats in your diet to active compounds which offer a natural protection against excessive water loss. Fatty acids are thought to be incorporated into the structural fatty compounds (phospholipids) of your skin, helping to normalize the fat layers by altering membrane fluidity. Just as there are certain required amino acids that your body doesn't produce, the fatty acids you need for the prevention of dry skin are also called "essential" because you don't manufacture them, you must eat them. Your body is incapable of making the starting materials for the production of essential fatty acids.

The importance of essential fatty acids for cosmetic use was first recognized in the 1930s when fatty acid deficiency was first related to dryness or roughness of skin and to the tendency towards eczema and itchiness. It was not conceivable at that time that a normal diet would be deficient in essential fatty acids. Although processed and hydrogenated foods are antagonists of essential fatty acid metabolism, such foods were not yet popular in the 1930s.

Fatty acids are also important in the structure of cell membranes. They are present in high concentration in the reproductive organs. One of the most important functions of fatty acids is that of acting as precursors of prostaglandins. A precursor is a forerunner—something that precedes and is the source of another substance. Prostaglandins have hormonelike activity. Specifically, they are fast-acting biological regulators which are produced by the body, when and where they are required. Each prostaglandin has a unique effect. Because the effects of prostaglandins are so short-lived, they must be produced constantly. Just as all necessary human protein can be produced from amino acids, or any word can be formed from the letters of the alphabet, so the prostaglandins can be made from polyunsaturated fatty acids—provided they are present.

Medical literature of 1940 vintage suggested that fatty acids could be applied topically to help in wound healing and to promote tissue repair. Another study from the same era showed that topical application in an ointment base improved skin conditions caused by poor diets and stress.

Some people use salad dressings for topical applications. One very popular skin-care book recommends mayonnaise. Cosmetic creams containing polyunsaturated fatty acids have appeared in the marketplace. Salad oils are often rancid; mayonnaise, if not homemade or purchased in a health store, contains additives. My favorite makeup remover and moisturizer for outer health is 100-percent pure extra virgin sesame oil supreme. My favorite source for polyunsaturated fatty acids for inner health is 100-percent pure hulled sesame seed supreme.

## OTHER NUTRIENT BENEFITS

Here are a few more bonuses of sesame:

- The lecithin in sesame transcends other lecithin sources (such as soybean lecithin), because it is in the form of an emulsifier, which is easier for the body to handle.

- Sesame is richer in iron than egg yolk.
- There is more potassium and phosphorus in sesame seeds than in bananas or orange juice.
- Sesame is a very low-allergy food.

### SESAME FOR THE LACTATING MOTHER

All over the world women are capable of producing enough milk, even when food consumption is inadequate. Regardless of diet, the quantity of protein in human milk remains constant. The protein percentage of milk from poorly nourished mothers is surprisingly high. Although protein quantity remains the same, a baby gains more weight when the mother's diet is supplemented with *quality* protein, often as sesame.

The amino acid methionine in mother's milk varies with the mother's intake, even though the overall *amount* of protein doesn't. This amino acid is not plentiful in too many foods, but there is more methionine in sesame than in any other food. Lactating women can improve the quality of the milk they produce by adding sesame to their own diet.

## SELECTION AND STORAGE

### THE SEED

It is essential to buy *hulled* sesame seeds for several reasons. Removal of the hull reduces the content of oxalic acid, located in the outer layer of the seed. Calcium oxalate is listed as a solid poison. When consumed in conjunction with calcium, calcium oxalate may be formed. Calcium oxalate consumption has been found to promote mineral depletion, which may result in urinary complications. Calcium oxalate can induce arthritis, gout, and severe allergic reactions, and yet, endless numbers of health-seeking devotees consume it, unaware that they are totalling 2,800 milligrams of calcium oxalate in every 3½ ounces of unhulled sesame seed.

In addition, the hull is an attractant for aflatoxins, dust, dirt, fragments of twigs, insect larvae and even rodent excretia. Like many outer coverings in nature, it appears that the hull was meant to keep out environmental hazards and protect the delicate internal seed.

The United States Department of Agriculture Handbook #456 is one of the few books that lists the value of hulled sesame seeds. Other handbooks listing food values include the hull of the sesame, thereby giving misleading calcium compositions.

Hulling serves to improve digestibility. Without the hull, sesame seeds are the most alkaline protein food known. But *caveat emptor:* The seeds should be hulled mechanically, without the use of chemicals. Some companies use a hot alkali, such as sodium hydroxide solution, to loosen or disintegrate the hulls. Then hydrochloric acid solution is used to neutralize the sodium hydroxide, leaving a residue of sodium chloride (salt).

It's not difficult to tell the difference between quality hulled sesame seeds and those that have been discredited with quick and caustic processing methods. Mechanically hulled sesame has a little black dot on the end of the seed. That black dot is the umbilicus, the site where the seed is attached to the pod. If that black dot is present, then you know that the seeds have not been subjected to chemical substances. These are the seeds you want to buy. In addition to the presence of the little black umbilicus, the seeds should be plump and should have color. Caustic substances flatten the shape of the seeds and bleach them white. Chemically hulled sesame seeds contain denatured protein and lipids, and decreased digestibility values. Mechanically hulled, chemical-free sesame seeds are free of aflatoxins and demonstrate a 99-percent reduced bacteria count compared to the unhulled seeds. When hulled properly, the seeds remain pure and sweet, and the unique antioxidant qualities are left intact. Mechanically hulled seeds will not turn rancid easily and will even remain fresh when stored at room temperature without refrigeration. Most important, the enzymes are intact.

## THE OIL

Every supermarket and grocery store sells refined, colorless sesame oil. This is the kind you should *not* buy—mainly because of the excessive use of high temperatures during processing of the seed for oil extraction and also because the oil has usually been *expressed* with the hulls.

The sesame oil you want to buy is 100-percent pure extra virgin supreme, extracted at low temperatures, without the use of chemical solvents such as hexane. Sesame oil requires very little refining. One reason that commercial companies resort to extreme refining measures is that they usually extract the oil from seeds with the hulls on. Quality sesame oil is taken from seeds that are hulled, of highest quality, chemical-free and very fresh.

Sesame is a tropical plant and therefore, nature has provided it with a much needed resistance to oxidation—the kind that takes place more easily at higher temperatures. Olive oil is an example of this too. Sesame has a lighter and fresher taste than olive oil. (Olive oil is monounsaturated. Sesame is polyunsaturated.)

Look for sesame oil that is produced in this country and doesn't have to be shipped from overseas. Remember that the higher the oil content of any product, the more quickly it becomes rancid. You don't want oil that has taken a long voyage or has to sit in a warehouse awaiting letters of credit or importation papers. It is virtually impossible to get olive oil in this country that does not have some degree of rancidity, but you can get sesame oil that is produced in the United States. Again—look for the bottle that says "100% Pure Extra Virgin Sesame Oil Supreme."

One of the reasons there is so much inferior sesame seed and oil on the market is that the small size of the seed makes hulling a difficult process. Fortunately, quality hulled seed and oil are available—products devoid of rancid hull fragments and overprocessing.

## RECIPES

Sesame has a variety of uses in food preparation. As stated, one of the advantages of sesame is its unusual amino acid profile. Because it is high in sulphur-containing amino acids in particular (which most other vegetable foods lack), it should be combined with wheat, rice, legumes or buckwheat to create more complete protein.

### IN SALADS: TASTY TOSSES

Sesame seeds must be chewed thoroughly to insure digestion. If not, they tend to go "right through," undigested. Therefore, sprinkle sesame seeds liberally on all of your crispy salads that require chewing—carrot salads, mixed raw vegetable salads and so on. (Use ground sesame or in butter form for dishes that are not chewy, such as yogurt or hot cereals.)

### AS TAHINI: MID-EAST MASTERY

Tahini is used in sauces and dressings, and as a spread. This is an excellent way to assimilate the nutrients found in sesame seeds, since we can't easily digest them unless they are physically broken down beforehand, or thoroughly chewed.

The much appreciated smooth taste of tahini has given rise to the saying, "to change the rough sea into taheen," meaning to smooth out all difficulties.

Food processing alters not only protein quantity, but the structural makeup of proteins as well. Researchers at the department of food science and technology at Oregon State University report that proteins are so delicate that mild treatment which does not change ordinary chemicals will affect protein. A raw egg has better protein quality than a cooked egg, and a lightly steamed egg has better protein quality than a hard-boiled egg, just as pure rare meat has superior protein when compared to meat that is well done. With animal products, however, care must be taken that raw or undercooked foods are not contaminated with or contain bacteria. Unheated sesame seeds are better for you than toasted sesame seeds. Tahini can be made from toasted or raw seeds. Although both are delicious, the toasted seeds lend an additional taste treat and aroma. The untoasted seeds contain more undisturbed nutrients. The choice is yours.

If you are going to heat sesame seeds, here are some tips. Heat a small, heavy skillet over medium heat and add hulled seeds. Stir and roast until seeds turn a few shades darker and you begin to smell that wonderful roasted scent. As the seeds roast, some will appear to be winged, and will fly out of your pan. Avoid fly-away losses by covering the pan with a mesh spatter-shield or strainer. If you want an exotic accoutrement in your kitchen, you can purchase a Japanese sesame-seed roaster. They are inexpensive and look like meshed wire boxes with handles. An opening at the top allows you to feed the seeds into the box. You simply hold the box over the heat on your stove and shake it.

Roasted seeds can be pulverized in an electric coffee grinder or a food processor, with a mortar and pestle, or even between two flat-bottomed ceramic plates. (Less seed is required for the mortar and pestle method.)

When using the electric grinder or food processor, stop the machine whenever the pastelike collection accumulates and slows things down. Use the other methods when you don't require complete pulverization. You may also purchase a Japanese grinder designed for the purpose. (They even have fine and coarse adjustments.)

**Sesame paste.** Roast and grind 3 tbsp of hulled sesame seeds. Add 1 tbsp of sesame oil slowly, mixing as you do so. Use to embellish any boiled or steamed vegetable.

**Tahini.** Heat a 7-inch skillet over medium heat. When hot, add one cup of hulled sesame seeds. Shake skillet until seeds are roasted. Pour seeds into blender or food processor. Begin blending and adding cold water at the same time. Stop adding water when paste is slightly thinner than peanut butter. This usually takes about 6 tablespoons of water. Homemade tahini will keep in the refrigerator for a week. It may also be frozen. Use as sauce or dip for raw vegetables.

**Tahini Lemon Sauce.** A more flavorful tahini sauce can be made with garlic and lemon juice. Crush 2 or 3 cloves of peeled garlic to a paste. Place in stainless steel or glass bowl. Add 1/4 cup tahini, and beat in with a fork. Add 4 tbsp lemon juice, beating as you do so. Add 3 tbsp cold water, just a little at a time, beating in as you go along. Amounts of garlic and lemon juice can vary according to taste. Use blender or food processor to avoid hand-beating. Add chopped parsley if desired.

## IN SAUCES: DRESSING FOR DINNER

Because sauces are not chewed, sesame seeds used for this application should always be ground.

**Sesame Dressing.** 1/4 cup ground sesame seeds; 1/2 cup water; 2 tbsp lemon juice; 1/2 clove garlic, crushed.

Blend all ingredients until smooth. Yields 3/4 cup dressing.

**Lemon Tahini Sauce.** 1 cup tahini; 2 cups water; juice of 2 lemons; 2 cloves garlic; 3 tbsp tamari soy sauce.

Blend ingredients. Warm gently and serve over fish.

**Green Goddess Dressing.** 1 1/2 very ripe, large avocados; 1 1/2 cups tahini; 4 cups water; 1 tbsp ground cumin; 2 tbsp fresh parsley.

Mash avocado. Mix tahini and water. Stir in avocado. Place in blender with remaining ingredients and blend until smooth.

**Sesame coating mix.** 1 cup whole wheat flour; 2 tbsp ground sesame seeds; 1 tbsp hulled sesame seeds; 1 tbsp dried parsley; 1 tsp dried oregano; 1 tsp garlic powder; 1 tsp paprika; 1/4 tsp cayenne pepper; 1/8 tsp ground cloves.

In bowl, combine all ingredients; mix well. Store in covered dish and refrigerate. Yields 1 1/2 cups. Use for poultry, fish and sliced vegetables. Place sesame coating mix in plastic food bag. Moisten food pieces with water; place a few pieces in bag; shake to coat evenly. Note: 1/2 cup of mix coats 2 1/2 lbs. chicken parts or 3 cups sliced vegetables.

## AS DINNER: THE MAIN COURSE

**Sesame Tofu Pilaf.** 3 cups cooked brown rice; 2 cups hulled sesame seeds; 3 blocks pressed tofu, diced; 1 small green pepper, diced; 3 scallions, diced; 1 cup bean sprouts; 1/2 tsp fresh minced ginger; 2 tsp fresh minced garlic; 2 tsp sesame oil; 2 tsp fresh minced parsley; tamari to taste.

Heat oil. Add garlic and ginger. Sizzle (do not brown). Add tofu, pepper, scallions, and gently sauté, adding tamari to taste. Stir in sprouts near completion. Separately mix sesame seeds with hot rice and sautéed ingredients into mix. Sprinkle in parsley. Top with tahini sauce.

**Vegetarian Meatloaf.** 1 cup hulled sesame seeds; 2 cups cooked brown rice; 1 cup millet; 1 cup bulgur wheat; 1 cup barley; 1 1/2 cups ground unsalted raw peanuts; 1/2 cup ground almonds; 1 1/2 cups tahini; 4 tbsp minced parsley; 2 tsp thyme; 2 tbsp chopped chives; 2 minced carrots; 2 minced celery stalks; 2 cups chopped mushrooms; 4 tbsp sesame oil; tamari to taste.

Preheat oven to 350°. Heat oil in skillet. Add vegetables; stir briefly. Add seasoning and tamari. Set aside in mixing bowl. Mix grain with nuts and seeds. Add tahini; blend well. (Tahini acts as natural binder.) Add vegetables. Lightly oil Pyrex dish and press mix into it. Bake 30 minutes.

## IN SOUPS: A MEAL IN A BOWL

**Cream of Carrot Soup.** 10 medium carrots, chopped; 2 stalks celery, chopped; 1 to 2 quarts water; 3 tsp garlic, minced; 1 1/2 cups tahini; 2 tbsp fresh parsley, minced; 1/4 cup unsalted cashew nuts, crushed; tamari to taste.

In large kettle, simmer vegetables in water until barely tender. Add garlic. In blender, puree soup. Add tahini and parsley. Blend thoroughly. Stir in cashew nuts and season to taste with tamari. Serve warm, but not boiling hot.

## IN ETHNIC DISHES: WORLDLY WONDERS

**Hummus.** 1-lb can garbanzo beans (chick peas); ¾ cup hulled sesame seeds; ½ cup water; juice of 1 lemon; 1 clove garlic, minced; 2 tsp dried parsley.

In saucepan gently heat beans in own water; drain and reserve liquid. Place seeds in blender with water and lemon juice. Blend to soft texture. Add garlic and parsley. Add warm beans a little at a time and blend at medium speed, stopping to stir mixture occasionally. When mixture churns steadily in blender, add bean liquid to adjust to desired consistency.

**Baba Ganouj.** 2 medium eggplants; 3 tbsp garlic, minced; 1 tbsp olive oil; 2 tbsp fresh parsley, minced; 1 cup tahini; 2 leaves fresh basil; 1 small onion, chopped.

Roast eggplants at 350° until soft. Remove skin; blend with remaining ingredients. Serve chilled as dip or salad on bed of raw spinach leaves with olives, peppers and pita bread wedges.

## IN CHILDREN'S FAVORITES: FUN FOODS (FOR KIDS OF ALL AGES)

**Sesame-peanut butter spread.** ½ cup sesame meal; ½ cup natural peanut butter; 1 ripe banana, mashed; sprinkle of currants.

Mix all ingredients. Enjoy plain, on sliced apples, or on rice cakes.

**Yogurt Delight.** ½ cup yogurt; 3 tsp ground sesame seed. Add to favorite fruit dishes.

**No-Bake Granola.** 1 cup sesame seeds; 2 tbsp sesame oil; 2 cups fine rolled oats; ¼ cup sprouted wheatberries; ½ cup chopped almonds; ½ cup sunflower seeds; ¼ cup pumpkin seeds; ½ cup unsweetened coconut meal; ½ cup chopped raisins.

Grind sesame seeds. Blend in oil. Add remaining ingredients, mixing thoroughly. Store in covered container in refrigerator. Serve with yogurt or juice. Add fresh fruit pieces if desired. Makes 5 to 6 cups granola.

**Hi-Protein Fruit Drink.** 1 cup fresh pineapple chunks; 4 ounces tofu; 1 tbsp tahini; 1 ripe banana.

Puree all ingredients in blender.

## AS OIL: FRIED RIGHT—LIGHT!

Sesame works well in salads and as a cooking oil, and it can be substituted for butter. Because the pure, virgin variety has a sweet taste, you will never miss butter. Use sesame oil to grease pans for grilling, especially for low temperature recipes.

You probably know that olive oil and safflower oil do not work for light frying. Sesame oil does. It is ideal for stir-frying. Because it is unrefined, sesame oil has a low boiling point, so it is not to be used when high temperatures are required. Note: High-temperature cooking is a method that is not in your best health interest under any conditions).

## AS PROTEIN COMPLEMENT: BALANCING AMINO ACIDS

**Morning cereal.** 1 part sesame seeds; 1 part millet; and 1 part wheatberries. Or substitute ½ measure of brewer's yeast for wheatberries. (Wheatberries should soak overnight. Even better, soak overnight, drain, and allow to sprout for 12 to 48 hours for additional nutrient value.)

Mix all three ingredients. The limiting amino acids of millet are tryptophan and lysine, but sesame supplies methionine. Sesame seeds need lysine, but supply methionine and tryptophan. Either wheatberries or brewer's yeast supply lysine, but require methionine and tryptophan.

**Seed snack.** 2 parts pumpkin seed; 1 part sesame seed; and 1 part wheatberries. (Soak wheatberries overnight. Optional: Allow wheatberries to sprout for 12 to 48 hours after soaking for additional nutrient value.)

Mix all three ingredients. Pumpkin seeds need methionine, but supply tryptophan. Sesame requires lysine, but offers methionine and tryptophan. Wheatberries supply lysine, but need the methionine and tryptophan.

**More seed snacks.** 3 parts sunflower seeds; 1 part sesame seeds; 2 parts wheatberries. (Soak wheatberries and sunflower seeds overnight. Optional: Sprout sunflower seeds 12 to 24 hours, and wheatberries 12 to 48 hours for additional nutrient value.)

Mix all three ingredients. Sunflower seeds require methionine and lysine, but do not offer any of the missing amino acids required by sesame or wheatberries. Sesame needs lysine, but supplies methionine and tryptophan. Wheatberries contain lysine, but require methionine and tryptophan.

## SUMMARY

Sesame is a good complementary source of protein and has an excellent fatty acid profile. It is high in methionine and tryptophan, which are limiting amino acids in many plant foods. Sesame's lysine content, although small in quantity, is highly stable. Vegetarians benefit from the special protein attributes of sesame. Soy flour protein can be improved by 100 percent with the addition of sesame. Even if you never eat sesame seeds except as a topping on a cracker, that cracker is considerably more nutritious because of the sesame topping.

# BREWER'S YEAST, WHEAT GERM AND OTHER HIGH POWER FOODS

*The Foods That Enrich You Nutritionally . . . What You Need to Know*

••

BEATRICE TRUM HUNTER

THE NUTRITIONAL GIANTS—HIGH POWER FOODS

Few of us eat such a good diet that we need no supplemental help to make it better. The exceptional foods described in this chapter are so powerful that they are needed only in modest amounts to reap great health benefits. The uses and functions of almost a dozen of these concentrated nutrients are discussed, such as the familiar vitamin B-complex powerhouse, brewer's yeast, and lecithin, cholesterol's enemy. For daily needs as well as in times of stress, this information can prove to be invaluable.

## WHY USE HIGH POWER FOODS?

Three important features of any good diet are variety, balance and moderation. If you adhere to these three features in selecting foods you won't go astray. Chances are good that you will reap health benefits.

What is the role, then, of high power foods? These substances should be regarded as supplements, used in addition to good foods, not to replace them. These concentrated nutrients can enhance good diets and make them even better. However, they will not turn a poor diet into a good one. At best, they may only be able to buffer some of the harm inflicted by a poor diet.

Some nutritionists have begun to classify foods according to their "nutrient density" scores, in terms of the ratio of nutrients to calories in individual foods. On this basis, foods such as turnip greens, parsley, bell pepper, collard greens, calf's liver and cantaloupe score high in their nutrients compared to their calories. At the other end of the scale, pecan pie, pretzels and gelatin dessert score low as classic "empty" calorie foods, being low in nutrients but high in calories.

The high power nutritional supplements selected to be discussed are all concentrated in nutrients. Therefore, you may benefit from these substances, if they are added in small amounts to the daily diet. Many of them are higher in phosphorus than calcium. For this reason, it is important to obtain adequate calcium, from foods and/or supplements, in order to balance the calcium-phosphorus ratio. Calcium is needed for the utilization of phosphorus; together they maintain healthy bones, proper metabolism, etc.

The compositions of most of the foods discussed are analyzed in Table 1.

## BREWER'S YEAST

Brewer's yeast, a one-cell plant, is about the size of a human blood corpuscle. Despite its diminutive size, brewer's yeast is a high power food. Food yeasts reproduce by putting forth successive buds that

TABLE 1. COMPOSITION OF SOME HIGH POWER FOODS*

| *ONE TABLESPOON OF:* | Grams | Calories g | Protein g | Fat g | Carbohydrates g | Calcium mg | Phosphorus mg | Iron mg | Sodium mg | Potassium mg | Vitamin A IU | Thiamin mg | Riboflavin mg | Niacin mg | Ascorbic acid mg |
|---|---|---|---|---|---|---|---|---|---|---|---|---|---|---|---|
| Brewer's yeast debittered | 8.0 | 23.0 | 3.1 | 0.1 | 3.1 | 17.0 | 140.0 | 1.4 | 10.0 | 152 | trace | 1.25 | 0.34 | 3.0 | trace |
| Sesame seeds, dry, dehulled | 8.0 | 47.0 | 1.5 | 4.3 | 1.4 | 9.0 | 47.0 | 0.2 | —** | — | — | 0.01 | 0.01 | 0.4 | 0 |
| Sunflower seeds, dry, dehulled | 9.1 | 50.8 | 2.2 | 4.3 | 1.8 | 10.9 | 75.9 | 0.64 | 2.75 | 83.4 | 4.4 | 0.18 | 0.02 | 0.49 | — |
| Pumpkin seeds, dry, dehulled | 8.8 | 48.4 | 2.5 | 4.1 | 1.3 | 4.4 | 100.1 | 0.98 | — | — | 6.3 | 0.02 | 0.02 | 0.21 | — |
| Wheat germ, toasted, without salt or sugar | 6.0 | 23.0 | 1.8 | 0.7 | 3.0 | 3.0 | 70.0 | 0.5 | trace | 57.0 | 10.0 | 0.11 | 0.05 | 0.3 | 1 |

*adapted from *Nutritive Value of American Foods, Agriculture Handbook No. 456.* Agricultural Research Service, USDA, 1975

**dash denotes lack of reliable data

separate from the parent cells and continue to grow. The budding process is extremely rapid.

Food yeasts are of worldwide importance. Vast quantities can be grown readily, without soil, in factories that require little space compared to land used for crops.[1] Food yeasts can thrive even when they are grown on waste products from canning plants or paper mills.

If the product label merely says yeast, you have no idea of the substance which has been used for growing the yeast. While all food yeasts are nutritious, they vary in quality and potency.

Certain phrases may appear on food yeast labels that offer useful information. Some yeasts are grown on strains of *Saccharomyces cerevisiae,* which are high-quality food sources such as molasses fortified with minerals, or cereal grain by-products from beer brewing. Other yeasts, grown on *S. fragilia,* from whey, a by-product from cheese making, are also of good quality but are lower in potency. Torula-type yeasts are grown on *Candida utilis,* from sugar recovered from wood during the manufacture of wood pulp cellulose. This, too, utilizes a by-product, from sulfite pulp paper waste. A large oil company has also used ethyl alcohol, a by-product of petroleum refining, for growing food yeasts. This process is less expensive than other yeast production, and much of this type of yeast is sold to food processors to be used as an ingredient in foodstuffs.

"Brewer's yeast" earned its name because it was a by-product of brewing. When grown especially for human consumption, it may be termed "primary yeast," or "nutritional yeast." All are food yeasts. If the word "debittered" appears on the label, it means that after the dried yeast has been washed free of beer, it is treated to eliminate its bitterness and make it more palatable.

Food yeasts are a rich source of nutrients. In composition, they may be as much as 50 percent protein, and protein of a good quality. They have a favorable balance of essential amino acids (although somewhat low in methionine). Yeasts are one of the richest sources of the B vitamins (except B12 which is now included in some brands of brewer's yeast). Yeasts are good sources of minerals and trace minerals, especially selenium and chromium. These two trace elements, notably lacking in highly processed foods, are present in yeast in forms that are safe and bioavailable. The chromium value of brewer's yeast is ten times greater than from other good sources such as calf's liver or wheat germ.[2] Yeasts are high in phosphorus. In order to keep a favorable calcium-phosphorus balance, some yeast producers add calcium to their products. If this is not done, it would be wise to add your own calcium source from food and/or supplements when you use yeast.

Food yeasts are sold in several forms: as powders, flakes and tablets. Powders are the most potent, so less needs to be used. Flakes dissolve more readily, especially in cold liquids, but more needs to be used. Tablets, the most expensive form, are also the least potent. However, for those who travel, or who dislike the taste of yeast, tablets may be the most convenient or acceptable form.

Live yeast in baking (leavening) yeast is rich in thiamin. If consumed live, it would rob thiamin from other foods and sweep the nutrient out of the body with the excreta. Once the yeast is heated by baking, it is inactivated, and the problem is eliminated. In dried brewer's yeast, which has no leavening power, there are no live cells. There is no interference with thiamin absorption. On the contrary, the brewer's yeast surrenders its own rich supply of thiamin and makes this nutrient available when the yeast is digested in the human stomach and upper intestine.

Who benefits from yeast? Many people do, and animals, too! Yeast is a concentrated food that is a good addition for persons who try to maintain an optimal diet. Since yeast is low in fat, carbohydrates, sodium and calories, these characteristics make it especially useful for weight-watchers, vegetarians, diabetics and hypoglycemics.

Yeast is rich in nucleic acids, including RNA, the cellular component that governs many vital processes including the rate of aging. RNA also controls many functional mechanisms. Yeast helps the body's glucose tolerance mechanism function properly.[3] This feature is important in the control of blood sugar level. If not functioning properly, a breakdown of this mechanism can lead to diabetes.

Judging from animal experiments, yeast may act as a cholesterol reducer. Rats were fed cholesterol and cholic acid as part of their diet in order to induce a cholesterol rise. When baker's or brewer's yeast, or yeast fractions were added to the diet, a rise of serum cholesterol in the animals was either partially or totally prevented. The degree of response depended on the level of yeast added: the more yeast, the greater the cholesterol blockage.[4]

Should anyone avoid yeast? A few people should. Yeast is high in nucleic acids that form purines. So gout sufferers should avoid yeasts. Persons who suffer from yeast infections (*Candida albicans*) also need to avoid all yeasts and fermented foods.

If you are introducing yeast into your diet, be aware that some beginners experience bloating and flatulence. You can minimize or avoid such discomfort if you begin with a small amount of yeast (less than a teaspoonful) taken several times each day on an empty stomach, mixed with acidic fruit juice.

People find various ways in which to render the taste of yeast palatable—or at least not disagreeable! Different brands have different flavors, so purchase small quantities at first, and sample them. Also, be prepared to experiment. Some people mix yeast with strong-flavored fruit juices such as grapefruit, grape or pineapple. Others use milk, tomato juice or water. Strong flavors, such as molasses or peanut butter, will mask the yeast taste so that yeast can be worked into baked bean casseroles, or into peanut butter spread. For a thick shake, mix yeast, milk, banana and molasses in an electric blender. Try yeast in homemade vegetable soups, adding it just before serving. The flavor of vegetable soups is *improved* by the addition of yeast. For years, commercial soup processors have used yeast for flavor enhancement purposes. Now they also use yeast to boost the flavor in low-sodium products,[5] and to increase moisture retention and add nutritional value to baked goods.[6]

Yeast is economical, with no waste. It has a long shelf life and does not require refrigeration. Store it in a tightly closed container that excludes light. Keep it in a cool dry place.

## LECITHIN

Lecithin (pronounced LE-si-thin) consists of waxy hygroscopic phosphatides (complex phosphoric ester lipides) containing phosphorus and the fatty acids choline and inositol. It is nature's principal emulsifier. Phosphatides are found in all living cells in both animals and vegetables. In our food supply, the highest concentrations are found in animal products such as eggs, meat and fish. Fresh egg yolks contain from 8 to 10 percent phosphatides. Although soybeans only contain from 0.3 to 0.6 percent, they are used as the source for commercial lecithin, since they are less expensive.[7]

Early medical investigations offered encouraging information about lecithin's values. In 1952, Francis M. Pottenger, Jr., M.D., and Bernard Krohn, M.D., reported that they were able to lower abnormally high serum cholesterol levels by adding lecithin to the human diet.[8] Ignored or decried by the medical establishment, the finding was, nevertheless, noted by other investigators.[9] Subsequently, lecithin was found to increase high-density lipoproteins.[10] It is known that these substances protect the cardiovascular system.

In the mid 1970s, brain researchers presented a startling finding indirectly involving lecithin. Neurotransmitters carry chemical signals to the brain and play vital roles in human emotional and physical behavior. Unusually low amounts of one neurotransmitter, acetylcholine, were thought to be the prime cause of tardive dyskinesia, and also involved in other conditions such as mania and memory loss. What was the lecithin connection?

Complete breakdown of lecithin by the process of hydrolysis yields two fatty acid molecules, plus one molecule each of glycerol, phosphoric acid and choline. One of the chemical precursors of acetylcholine is the nutrient choline, and the major source of choline is lecithin.

In the early investigations, brain researchers used choline in both animal and human studies. They were able to raise the acetylcholine level to some degree. However, their results were better when they used lecithin mixed with puddings or other foods. By stimulating greater production of the brain's neurotransmitter, acetylcholine, they could suppress the tardive dyskinesia symptoms to a greater extent. It was thought that lecithin was more effective since, unlike pure choline, much of the lecithin is not broken down by bacteria in the intestine.[11]

Additional studies using lecithin have been made with senile dementia (Alzheimer's disease) and other neurological disorders.[12] When lecithin was supplied in an active form, in sufficient amounts, results were promising. However, most commercially available lecithin preparations contain low levels of choline, estimated to be from 2 to 4 percent. As a result, such preparations, labeled "pure," provided too little choline to stimulate acetylcholine formation or to improve disease states involving diminished acetylcholine release.[13]

"Lecithin is a word that health-conscious consumers have positive associations with," food processors were advised in a trade journal. "That's something to think about because the appearance of the label has a lot to do with any product's success in the market—or even in getting to the market."[14] Food processors have long been aware of lecithin's favorable image as well as its usefulness in food manufacture. In addition to functioning as an emulsifier, lecithin acts as an anti-sticking agent, a wetting and dispersing agent, and an antioxidant.

Commercial soybean lecithin is a mixture of three phospholipids dissolved in soybean oil which is used as a carrier. Formerly, the commercial product consisted of 62 to 70 percent phospholipids and 30 to 38 percent associated soybean oil and vegetable fatty acids. At present, food processors can choose from several grades of lecithin, including an oil-free powder, fine or large granules, and a special modified water-dispersable product.

Lecithin that is separated from soybean oil is known as "crude lecithin" or "commodity-grade lecithin." "Lecithin concentrates" are products in a thick liquid state. They are mixtures of phosphatides from the soybean oil and some residual oil as a carrier.[15] Three types of concentrates are available. One concentrate has a light brown color and is an unbleached fluid that pours at room temperature. Another is as thick as most liquid lecithins but has a higher activity and contains no fatty acids. It is stable and has less tendency than other liquid lecithins to thicken with long storage or under moist conditions. The third type is a fluid that has been bleached twice to reduce its color to a light amber.[16]

"Lecithin granules" are processed phosphatides. Most products are extracted with acetone, a solvent, that is then removed and reused. If lecithin granules dissolve in water, this signifies that they have been acetone-extracted.

In addition to its many food applications, lecithin is useful in cosmetics and pharmaceuticals. Also, there are numerous industrial uses: paints, printing inks, gasoline, lubricating oils and other petroleum products. Synthetic forms are dimyristoyl, dipalmitoyl, distearoyl and dioleoyl lecithin.[17]

As a food supplement, lecithin is available in three forms: granules, capsules and liquid. Granules are mild-flavored and agreeable, even when eaten from a spoon. You can sprinkle them over foods such as cereals or casseroles, mix them in juices or soups, or add them to baking dough or pancake batter. The capsules are useful for travel but their potency is lower. About ten 1200-milligram capsules equal the amount of lecithin in one tablespoon of the granules. Liquid lecithin consists of about two-thirds lecithin and one-third soybean oil. The oil adds calories. For many people, the texture of the thick liquid as well as its flavor makes it unpalatable to be used "neat." However, liquid lecithin can replace some cooking or baking oil or fat. If you spread a small quantity of liquid lecithin into baking pans you can achieve a non-stick coating. The baked goods will slide out readily and the pans will clean easily.

After you open containers of granules or tablets, close them tightly and store in a cool dry place. The granules have a relatively long shelf life, but in time, they become dry and rubbery in texture. Since liquid lecithin contains oil, refrigerate it after the container is opened.

## SESAME, SUNFLOWER AND PUMPKIN SEEDS

The old saw that "good things come in small packages" certainly applies to edible seeds. Despite their size, all seeds store concentrations of nutrients, held in readiness for reproduction and development of the new plant.

Among edible seeds, sesame, sunflower and pumpkin have high nutritional ratings. In 1961, farmers were advised by USDA in its yearbook on seeds, that for planting purposes, a pound of sesame seeds contained 150 thousand; a pound of sunflower seeds, 10.4 thousand; and a pound of pumpkin seeds, between 1.6 and 4.8 thousand. At that time, farmers had valued such seeds for the production of oil and for by-products used in animal feed. Until relatively recently only a small subculture of health-minded individuals and people in Eastern cultures recognized the nutrient offerings from such seeds. For most people, sesame seeds were merely the garnishes on rolls, and sunflower or pumpkin seeds, the "polly seeds" for birds.

The situation has changed, however. Many people now recognize sesame seeds as a nutritious food that can make a contribution to the diet. Sunflower and pumpkin seeds have become widely recognized in snack foods, granola-type cereals, and even in nationally distributed bread. Now that packets of sunflower or pumpkin seeds are sold at bus terminals, railway stations and airports, truly it can be said that these seeds have arrived!

"Open sesame" is a well-deserved metaphor for splendor and richness. The sesame plant may have originated long ago, in Africa and then spread to India, China and Japan. Its antiquity is revealed in Assyrian tablets, and Babylonian records mention the importance of this seed for ceremonies, herbal medications and wine.

Sesame was grown primarily for its oil content, which is still valued for its stability, color, flavor and resistance to rancidity. In early civilizations, sesame was not used as food, for the traditional wisdom held that the hull was unhealthy. This belief was correct. Although the hull contains calcium, it also contains a high level of toxic calcium oxalate crystals.[18] Oxalates, consumed at high levels, interfere with calcium absorption and may lead to numerous health problems.[19] The only means of removing the hull was by hand rubbing, a laborious and unsatisfactory procedure.

In recent times, it became technically feasible to remove the hull by means of chemical treatments, using caustic lye along with calcium carbonate, neutralizing acids, salts, bleach and high drying temperature. These harsh treatments were undesirable, since contact of the sesame seed, even briefly, with such substances profoundly damages the quality of the protein and the oil and makes the oil turn rancid quickly.

Fortunately, a technique has been perfected to dehull the sesame seed without resorting to harsh, damaging treatments. Seeds dehulled mechanically, not chemically, are available, with a statement of this method noted on the labels.

Dehulled whole sesame seeds can be sprinkled over cereals, soups and casseroles; added to bread dough and pancake batter; combined with confection ingredients; and, of course, used as a garnish. Sesame seeds can be ground into meal in an electric seed grinder or with a mortar and pestle. "Gomasia," a seasoning, is a mixture of sesame meal and sea salt. "Tahini," finely ground sesame seeds, is a spread similar to peanut butter. Tahini, mixed with honey, makes "Halvah," a popular Near Eastern confection. Or, blended with water, tahini makes a sesame "milk" that serves as a base for fruit drinks; mixed with oil and vinegar, it is turned into salad dressing.

Dehulled whole sesame seeds, as well as sesame meal, should be stored in a cool dry place, in tightly closed containers that exclude air. Once the containers have been opened, sesame products should be refrigerated.

Sunflower seeds, too, are storehouses of concentrated nutrients.

Since native Americans worshipped the sun, they esteemed the sunflower as it followed the sun's movement, heliotropically through the daylight hours. Native Americans used sunflower seeds in a variety of ways in their diet. It is believed that sunflower oil, now commonly used in parts of Europe, was introduced to the Old World by Spaniards who carried it from the area that is now New Mexico.

We have become the world's largest exporter of sunflower seeds. The growth has been spectacular. Our production expanded from 0.5 million metric tons in 1976-1977 to 3.5 million tons in 1979-1980. Our share of world production, less than 3 percent in 1974-1975, soared to 25 percent in 1979-1980. Our tremendous growth in production was accomplished by a 440 percent increase of sunflower crop acreage, as well as a 35 percent growth in average crop yield.[20] About 25 percent of the sunflower seed's value is derived from the meal, and about 75 percent from the oil. Sunflower oil now competes with corn and safflower oils. It is higher in polyunsaturates than corn oil. When heated, sunflower oil is more stable than safflower oil.

Dehulled sunflower seeds can be eaten as they are, and make an excellent snack. They can be used in many ways already described for sesame seeds. A unique feature is that even after the hulls have been removed from sunflower seeds, they are still viable and will sprout. Sunflower seed sprouts taste best when the sprouts are only about a quarter of an inch long.

Pumpkins seeds, too, are concentrated in nutrients, and make a good snack. Pumpkin seeds have been esteemed in folk medicine as a treatment for various ailments. In the mid-1800s, pumpkin seeds were listed in the U.S. Pharmacopoeia as a diuretic as well as a worm remedy.[21] Pumpkin seeds have been held in high regard by many groups as a folk remedy for prostate problems. Modern medicine may confirm this feature. It happens that pumpkin seeds are good sources of magnesium and zinc, and frequently both minerals are recommended as supplements in prostate therapy.

## WHEAT AND CORN GERMS

In milling grain, the embryo of the kernel is removed to prevent rancidity in the flour. If you use *freshly* ground whole grain flour, the germ will be in the flour and it will not be rancid.

If you choose to buy wheat germ separate from the flour, make certain that the product is fresh, for wheat germ is among those foods that turn rancid rapidly. Ideally, the product should be vacuum-packed. If not, it should be refrigerated and bear either a packing or end date on the label. After you open the container, transfer the contents to a strong paper bag, inserted in a plastic bag. Fold both bags down tightly to exclude air as much as possible. Store the bag in the refrigerator, or better still, in the freezer. Wheat germ is free flowing, and even when it is taken directly from the freezer, it is not caked.

Some controversy exists as to whether one should eat wheat germ raw or toasted. The toasting helps retard rancidity. Both forms are nutritious. You can sprinkle wheat germ over cereals, soups and casseroles; add it to bread dough and pancake batter; and mix it with meat, fish or poultry loaves or patties.

Corn germ is less well known but has been available since a method was devised to stabilize its fat. The corn germ is a valuable source of vitamin B and minerals. It contains more lysine than whole-kernel corn, and it may be second only to beef liver as an excellent source of iron.[22] Corn germ has a pleasant texture, popcorn-like flavor, and is more stable than wheat germ. It can be added to baked goods, granola-type cereals, stuffings and casseroles.

## REFERENCES

1. Gerard, Ralph W., Ph.D., M.D., ed. 1952. *Food for Life.* Chicago, IL: University of Chicago Press
2. *Journal of Agricultural & Food Chemistry,* January/February 1973

3. *Modern Medicine,* September 16, 1974; *Medical World News,* October 11, 1974
4. *Journal of Food Science,* May/June 1977
5. *Snack Food,* October 1980; *Food Processing,* June 1975
6. *Baking Industry,* February 1978
7. *Food Engineering,* November 1981
8. *Journal of Digestive Diseases,* April 1952
9. *Australian & New Zealand Journal of Medicine,* June 1977; *Clinical Research,* Vol. 25, No. 2, 1977; *Current Therapeutic Research,* August 1978
10. *Nutrition & Metabolism,* Vol. 17, No. 6, 1974
11. *Science News,* February 11, 1978
12. *New York Times,* January 26, 1978; *Science News,* December 12, 1981
13. *The Professional Nutritionist,* Summer 1979
14. *Food Development,* November 1981
15. *Food Processing,* November 1981
16. *Food Plant Ideas,* June 1979
17. *Science* [advertisement] November 28, 1980
18. *American Journal of Clinical Nutrition,* October 1973
19. *Journal of the Irish Medical Association,* February 22, 1975
20. *National Food Review,* Fall 1980
21. Friedlander, Barbara. 1974. *The Secrets of the Seed Vegetables, Fruits & Nuts.* New York, NY: Grosset & Dunlap
22. *Food Product Development,* August 1980

# Caprenin: It's Low-Fat But How Safe Is It?

In response to current recommendations to reduce dietary fats—especially saturated fats—some manufacturers are reformulating candy bars, using caprenin as a cocoa butter replacer. Caprenin is composed of naturally occurring fatty acids, mainly behemic acid, as well as caprylic and capric acids. Hydrogenated rapeseed (canola), coconut and palm kernel oils are used as sources for caprenin.

Caprenin has similar properties to cocoa butter, but it has only five calories per gram, compared with nine calories per gram in other fats. The reason that caprenin is lower in calories is because behemic acid is absorbed only partially by the body and capric and caprylic acids are metabolized less efficiently than other fatty acids.

Procter & Gamble commissioned FASEB (*Federation of American Societies for Experimental Biology*) to review caprenin's safety, in order to petition the FDA to grant it GRAS (*Generally Recognized as Safe*) status. The experts judged that caprenin is digested, absorbed and metabolized by the usual pathways. However, they reocmmended that a toll-free number be listed on labels of products containing caprenin. The reason, according to one FASEB panelist, Professor Bert La Du, Jr., "is the lack of real experience in people with a compound that is new, and to be sure that if anything were missed in the review, there is an easy way for people . . . to report any adverse findings. No matter how much anmal testing, until you have human experience, it isn't possible to judge what the experience will be." Similar concern was raised by another panelist, Dr. Elaine B. Feldman, who urged that "we ought to learn more about the effects of ingesting it because it is an artificial substance."

By late 1994, the concerns were justified. In reviewing the safety data to affirm caprenin as GRAS, the FDA expressed concern regarding "possible implications for human safety," involving liver damage from long-term caprenin ingestion. Liver enzyme levels, espeically GPT (glutamic-pyruvic transaminase) were beyond the normal range in some humans consuming caprenin. Increased liver enzyme activities were observed in rats in both short-term (28 days) and long-term (90 days) feeding studies, as well as in short-term (5 days) human clinical trials. Repeated and/or continued gastrointestinal distress was noted. Also, caprenin consumption increased total cholesterol, low-density lipoprotein cholesterol, and the ratio of total cholesterol to high-density lipoprotein cholesterol. Although GRAS status for caprenin is pending, its use in candy bars continues and its expanded use by food processors with wider applications is a likely development.

BEATRICE TRUM HUNTER

# LIPOIC ACID: THE METABOLIC ANTIOXIDANT

*The Unique Nutrient That Recharges Energy Levels and the Body's Defenses*

RICHARD A. PASSWATER, PH.D.

THE ULTIMATE PARTNER

Unlike other valuable antioxidants, lipoic acid is both water- and fat-soluble, so can be used throughout the body. It enhances the effect of other antioxidants and helps them resist being used up as they defend the body against free-radical damage. This concise but comprehensive guide shows how lipoic acid is effective against diabetes, heart disease and toxic metals, and even shows action against the HIV virus that causes AIDS.

## WHY ALL THE EXCITEMENT?

Scientists who study nutrition are very excited today about a once obscure nutrient, lipoic acid. What is lipoic acid and why all the excitement? Lipoic acid is a key compound for producing energy in muscles and an important link in the vital antioxidant network. It is an essential "key" that unlocks the energy from food calories. Lipoic acid directs calories into energy production and away from fat production. The energy produced is available not only for moving the skeletal muscles, but for everything we need to do. When we improve our efficiency to produce energy, we improve our ability to perform at top level in everything we do from exercising to thinking.

Lipoic acid normalizes blood sugar levels and reduces glycation, the damage sugar does to critical body components. This damage leads to accelerated aging, heart disease and the adverse effects of diabetes.

Although there are hundreds of studies over forty years revealing how lipoic acid energizes metabolism, the new excitement about this nutrient can be seen in the many recent studies focusing on how it improves the physique, combats free radicals, protects our genetic material, slows aging, helps protect against heart disease, cancer and many other diseases.

Both insulin-dependent and non-insulin dependent diabetics will be excited to learn that lipoic acid has been used for nearly thirty years in Europe to treat diabetic neuropathy, help regulate blood sugar, and prevent diabetic retinopathy and cardiopathy. Lipoic acid not only protects the nervous system, but may be involved in regenerating nerves as well. It is also being studied in the treatment of Parkinson's disease and Alzheimer's disease.

Lipoic acid has also been used for decades to protect the liver and to detoxify the body of heavy metal pollutants. One of the most exciting recent developments is that lipoic acid appears to help slow the progression of HIV infection to clinical AIDS. This is important not only to HIV-positive people, but to all of us, as AIDS treatment adds billions of dollars to our health costs which we all pay either as increased insurance premiums or taxes.

We make some lipoic acid in our bodies, but usually not enough, so we depend on food to get what we need for optimal health. This means that it is not quite a vitamin by definition, but is classified as the very next thing to a vitamin. Lipoic acid is also a "conditionally essential" antioxidant nutrient. Conditionally essential simply means that it is essential to life, but that young healthy people normally don't have to get all of it from food. Since our ability to make lipoic acid in our bodies tends to decline with age or disease, many people don't produce enough and their health becomes very dependent on how much they get in their diet.[1]

Lipoic acid's antioxidant function is of major imortance. Antioxidant nutrients help protect the body against the damage that can cause heart disease, cancer, aging and about eighty other diseases. This damage is caused by undesirable by-products of metabolism called free radicals. Not only does lipoic acid improve metabolism, it protects us against the harmful by-products of metabolism.

Lipoic acid both interacts with its antioxidant partners, vitamin E and vitamin C, and helps conserve them. When the body is deficient in lipoic acid, the other antioxidants do not properly network together.

Lipoic acid also protects the liver and detoxifies tissues of heavy metals such as excessive iron and copper, and the toxic metals cadmium, lead, and mercury.[2]

It is amazing that a single nutrient has so many actions. The value of lipoic acid to our health is best described by its nickname: the metabolic antioxidant. Lipoic acid is a coenzyme that is involved in metabolism (energy production) and a universal antioxidant that directly and indirectly helps protect every body component from the damage of oxidative stress.

## A DUAL HISTORY—METABOLISM AND ANTIOXIDANT

As long ago as 1951, lipoic acid attracted the interest of scientists who specialized in elucidating the roles of B-complex vitamins, because of its action as an essential coenzyme. A coenzyme is a nonprotein substance that combines with a protein to form a complete enzyme. An enzyme is a protein that speeds up reactions or makes it possible for certain reactions to occur in the body. Enzymes are not consumed in the reactions that they facilitate. Most human coenzymes are produced from some of the B-complex vitamins or are themselves vitamins.

At one time, lipoic acid seemed to be a member of the vitamin B complex. Lipoic acid seemed to be destined to become the first fat-soluble vitamin B isolated. But, as I noted earlier, lipoic acid is not a "true" vitamin because the body can make enough to prevent a recognizable deficiency disease (though not enough to perform all its functions, hence its "conditionally essential" status). As a coenzyme, lipoic acid has an advantage over most true vitamins, which have to be converted into coenzymes.[3]

Early clues to the function of lipoic acid suggested that it was a catalyst with high biological activity required for the oxidation of carbohydrates and fatty acids which leads to the generation of adenosine triphosphate (ATP). A catalyst is an element or compound that facilitates a reaction that might not otherwise occur to a significant extent without its help. Enzymes are catalysts that the body needs to carry out the thousands of biochemical reactions in the body needed for controlling the life process.[4]

The generation of ATP is critical. ATP is the compound that stores energy in the body. Energy is a force, not a compound, but energy can be stored in various ways, physically and chemically. The body stores energy in ATP and then releases when it's needed.

## LIPOIC ACID THE ANTIOXIDANT

It was realized fairly early that lipoic acid also served as a biological antioxidant when researchers found that it prevented scurvy in vitamin C deficient animals, and by 1988 it began to emerge as a universal antioxidant with many properties.

After the original flurry of research on lipoic acid as a coenzyme, interest faded when it looked doubtful that it was dietarily essential. Eventually it was noted that lipoic acid entered into a relationship with glutathione that protected cell components against lipid peroxidation. This was discovered by Drs. A. Bast and G. Haenen in 1988.[6,7]

Dr. Lester Packer of the University of California at Berkeley is a pioneer in the research on lipoic acid as an antioxidant. In 1991, he found it to be an important part of a network of antioxidants that includes vitamin C, vitamin E and glutathione. In 1993, Dr. Packer found that lipoic acid also functions to protect a key nuclear factor that is involved in the expression and regulation of genes. This has major implications for our health and will be discussed in detail later.[1]

Thus, the metabolic antioxidant, lipoic acid is multifunctional. It is essential for energy production, and provided enough is available in the body, it can act as a powerful antioxidant.

The chemical structure of lipoic acid is discussed in Appendix C.

## THE METABOLIC ENERGIZER

The energy needed to run our bodies actually comes from the energy of the sun that has been stored in food. Plants capture the sun's energy through a process called photosynthesis. This process combines sun energy with water and carbon dioxide to make carbohydrate, proteins and fats, also releasing oxygen to the air in the process. We, and other animals, breathe in the oxygen and eat plant food, and reverse this process. We convert food back into carbon dioxide, water and energy.

We need to metabolize energy from food for all of our life processes—everything from breathing to digestion to thinking to moving muscles. Metabolism is the process of life. It involves the breaking down of dietary carbohydrates, proteins and fats into smaller units, reorganizing these units as sources of energy, larger molecules and tissue building blocks, and eliminating waste products of the process. Lipoic acid is concerned with the catabolic portion of metabolism that breaks down the larger molecules (such as glycogen) into smaller molecules such as pyruvic acid. Specifically, lipoic acid is a key factor in converting food carbohydrates and fats into blood sugar (glucose) and fatty acids which then go through a process that leads to the extraction of energy. Lipoic acid is also involved in protein metabolism, but this is not a major energy pathway.

The body needs to "burn" blood sugar to produce energy, but instead of using high temperatures like those of a fire, the body has special biological catalysts called enzymes which extract the energy from sugars and fatty acids at normal body temperatures. Catalysts are atoms or molecules that facilitate reactions that either, as is the situation in the body, would not occur to any significant degree without their help, or in the case of commercial plant production, need to be sped up to be economically feasible. Catalysts are not consumed in these reactions, and a small amount can facilitate many cycles of the reaction that they facilitate.

Enzymes are proteins that act as catalysts and are not consumed in the process. They are there to facilitate the process along the way. As mentioned earlier, enzymes are made from coenzymes which in turn are often made from vitamins. Lipoic acid is a coenzyme that does not need a vitamin precursor.

Lipoic acid is a coenzyme for several key enzymes involved in energy production.

In essence, the body forms a multienzyme complex involving lipoic acid to break down molecules of pyruvate produced in earlier metabolism, into slightly smaller, high-energy molecules called acetyl-coenzyme A (acetyl-CoA). This results in molecules that can enter into a series of reactions called the citric acid cycle or Krebs cycle, which finishes the conversion of food into energy.

Sugars and fats are first harshly oxidized in the body by other enzymes that combine them with oxygen that we have breathed in through our lungs. These products must then be acted upon by the lipoic acid enzyme complex in order for the process to continue into the citric acid cycle.

Lipoic acid is involved in what is called a decarboxylation, which simply means that it cleaves off carbon dioxide. In the process excess energy is liberated which the body captures as ATP and then uses that to provide the energy for muscle contraction.

Lipoic acid is a cofactor in a multienzyme complex that catalyzes what biochemists like to call "oxidative decarboxylation of alpha-keto acids," such as pyruvic acid. Forget the jargon and just remember that pyruvic acid is a product of a process called glycolysis, which is the first step in converting blood sugar (glucose) into energy that the body can burn. The lipoic acid itself, a coenzyme, is bound to a very complex enzyme which is a high molecular weight protein and as such it is not consumed when it is serving as a metabolic cofactor but it is continually regenerated.

The metabolic function of lipoic acid occurs inside cells. The processes that it catalyzes actually occur in the round and rod-shaped structures called mitochondria in the cytosol (interior) of cells. Mitochondria are sometimes called the "powerhouse" of the cell, where food is converted into energy.

In 1984, a Dr. Reuben reported a clinical condition resulting from abnormal lipoic acid coenzyme function. This condition gives us a "tool" for determining what would happen in a lipoic acid deficiency. Dr. Reuben described the hypotonia (reduced solute concentration), failure to thrive, reduced muscle mass, cerebral cortical atrophy and severe lactic acid accumulation caused by this disorder. Lipoic acid supplementation relieved these problems.

In 1990, Dr. L. Yoshida and colleagues at the University of California at San Diego reported that lipoic acid supplementation benefited a patient with defective enzymes of the multienzyme complex.

The reason for going through all this biochemistry is to make sure three "take-home" messages are clear. First, a shortage of lipoic acid would be a critical bottleneck slowing down the energy process. If a person lacks energy because of a deficiency in lipoic acid, supplemental lipoic acid will restore that person's energy level to normal. However, lipoic acid is not a stimulant like caffeine.

## BLOOD SUGAR CONTROL

The second "take-home" message is that since lipoic acid facilitates the conversion of blood sugar into energy, it can have an effect on blood sugar level. Normally it is not the controlling factor for blood sugar level, because this entire process is subject to other types of enzymatic control. However, there is strong evidence that high intake of lipoic acid does influence glucose level. The high intake means a level that the body normally doesn't produce. This would be an effect of either diet or supplementation. It takes a consumption of more than 100 milligrams (preferably 500 to 600 milligrams) per day before any effect would be seen on glucose metabolism. Later on I discuss the research and experience gained through two decades of therapeutic use in Germany in the reduction of side effects in diabetes.

## GLYCATION

The third message is that lipoic acid supplements which normalize blood sugar levels also reduce glycation. Glycation is the process in which proteins react with excess glucose. This sugar damage is just as detrimental to protein as is oxygen damage. There is strong evidence that lipoic acid does keep the glucose level in the blood under control, and reduced levels of glucose mean less glycation. That is important in slowing aging and reducing diabetic side effects. The role of glycation in aging will be discussed in the section on aging.

## ENERGY AND PHYSIQUE ENHANCEMENT

For many of those with impaired energy production due to lipoic acid shortage, age or disease, supplementation may help restore the energy level to normal. Studies involving diabetics have shown that lipoic acid increases the amount of blood sugar converted into energy while not increasing the amount of blood sugar converted into fat.

When people have their energy level restored, then they can exercise harder and longer. With increased exercise, there is increased muscle growth and more mitochondria to burn food calories and build muscle. Increased muscle size increases the basic metabolic rate, which in turn decreases body fat. Lipoic acid can thus have a favorable effect on body structure by promoting increased muscle size and decreased body fat.

## SUMMARY

The three important messages in this section are:

1. Lipoic acid deficiency can be a bottleneck slowing energy production.
2. Lipoic acid supplementation can help normalize blood sugar levels. This is extremely important to diabetics.
3. Lipoic acid supplementation reduces glycation, which damages proteins and accelerates aging.

## PROTECTION AGAINST DISEASE

Lipoic acid's role as an outstanding, universal antioxidant is exciting many researchers today. The interest is so great because antioxidants help protect us from approximately 80 different age-related diseases. These diseases are not really caused by the mere passage of time, but by the cumulative damage done by free radicals to cell membranes and DNA.

It is becoming difficult to keep track of all the diseases that are now linked to free radicals. Free radicals are highly reactive entities that occur in the body and do damage that leads to disease. The list of free-radical related diseases reads like the table of contents of a general medical text. A 1993 study by Pracon, Inc., of Reston, Virginia, concluded that if Americans took optimal amounts of just the three best known antioxidant nutrients—beta-carotene, vitamin C and vitamin E—we would save $8.7 billion annually from reduced hospitalizations for heart disease and cancer alone.

These free radical diseases include cancer, heart attacks, strokes, rheumatoid arthritis, cataracts, and Alzheimer's disease—the major cause of admission to nursing homes. The list keeps growing. Before Dr. Denham Harman's "free radical theory of aging," disease was mostly attributed to germs and aging—and aging was an unknown process. Although Dr. Harman's theory of free radicals and aging was developed in 1956, it wasn't until years later that other researchers linked other diseases to free radicals (e.g., cancer by Passwater in 1972 and heart disease by Steinberg in 1981). Now we have disease pathologies involving free radicals that can be studied—and prevented, with the help of antioxidant nutrients such as lipoic acid.

It took a long while for the concept that free radicals could cause disease to be accepted. But it was also a long time before Louis Pasteur's germ theory was widely approved. A free radical is just as deadly as a germ, but in a different way. Of course, neither one germ nor one free radical presents a grave danger by itself. When germs infect a person—which usually happens only when their immune system is not functioning optimally—the germs (microorganisms such as viruses or bacteria) multiply and take over host functions. Free radicals also multiply and create chain reactions, and they do damage over time that alters body function.

Just as the wonder drugs—the antibiotics such as penicillin—cure killer infectious diseases, the wonder antioxidant nutrients can prevent killer diseases and help alleviate the symptoms and side effects of inflammatory diseases such as arthritis and even diabetes.

Antioxidant nutrients protect us from so many diseases because so many diseases involve free radicals and reactive oxygen species. Free radicals are molecules or fragments of molecules that are unstable and highly reactive. They are produced as the result of a normal molecule losing or gaining an electron.

In stable molecules, electrons normally associate in pairs. However, body processes such as metabolism can short-circuit the customary biochemical pathway, resulting in oxygen compounds that have lost an electron. This leaves each of these oxygen atoms or oxygen-containing molecules with an extra unpaired or lone electron. This is an oxygen free radical. Since the laws of nature work to restore atoms and molecules to their normal states, this oxygen atom becomes very reactive and seeks to regain an electron by grabbing one from another atom or molecule.

Several different types of oxygen radicals and other reactive oxygen species can be formed during normal metabolism. The table below lists the main oxygen radicals and reactive species. The hydroxyl radical is the most damaging radical to body components.

There are tens of thousands of free radicals created in the body every second. Critical body components such as DNA, the genetic material that directs the manufacture of each of our cells, can be altered by free radicals. The DNA in each cell may be hit about 10,000 times a day, according to Dr. Bruce Ames.

When one free radical captures an electron from another molecule, this creates a new free radical, as the second molecule now has a lone, unpaired electron. Of course, this new free radical will seek to capture another electron and become normal again. As you can see, this process could be never-ending. A free radical grabs electrons from anther molecule, which then becomes a free radical and grabs another electron from still another molecule, and on and on—a chain reaction. Some of the compounds are altered by this process and portions of DNA or cell membranes are damaged. As a result, they don't function properly and health is impaired.

Unfortunately, free radical chain reactions can take place in your body countless times a day. To make matters worse, there are other sources of free radicals besides those generated during oxygen metabolism. Cigarette smoke, pollutants, sunlight, radiation, and even emotional stress can create free radicals and cause free-radical chain reactions.

Fortunately, you have powerful defenses against these free radicals. If you nourish your body properly, you can make ample quantities of antioxidant enzymes that will terminate these free radical reactions. Your main antioxidant enzyme defenses are superoxide dismutase, catalase and glutathione peroxidase. These antioxidant enzymes require trace minerals including selenium, manganese, copper, zinc and iron.

Your body also relies directly on other nutrients that are themselves antioxidants to terminate free-radical reactions. Antioxidant nutrients have the ability to surrender electrons to rampaging free radicals without adding to the chain reaction. Thus, antioxidants can terminate reactive free radicals and, in turn, the antioxidant does not become a damaging free radical but a very sedate, low-energy, long-lasting free radical that does no further harm to the body. Such antioxidant nutrients include vitamin A, vitamin C, vitamin E, mixed carotenoids, bioflavonoids and lipoic acid.

Dr. Lester Packer has elucidated the mechanisms responsible for the synergism of the major antioxidant nutrients. It turns out that there are antioxidant cycles, in which one antioxidant can regenerate or recharge another that has been altered in a free radical reaction and can no longer function as antioxidant. Each antioxidant does not necessarily act on its own, but often antioxidants have interconnected actions, which determine the antioxidant potency of the body or parts of the body. In the case of the redox-based antioxidants like the thiols (including the glutathione and lipoic acid systems), the vitamin C system and the vitamin E antioxidant cycle, there is clearly a synergism that exists when all three components are interacting with one another.

When a compound is reduced, it gains an electron. When a compound is oxidized, it loses an electron. Reducing power refers to a compound's ability to donate an electron, that is, to reduce another compound. If a compound donates an electron easily, it has high reducing power. If it hangs on tightly to electrons, it has low reducing power.

Lipoic acid has a low redox potential, which means that its reduced form, dihydrolipoic acid, very readily donates electrons to other compounds.[8] So, for example, it can reduce oxidized glutathione to reduced glutathione. It also directly reduces the vitamin E radical, formed when vitamin E quenches lipid peroxidation, back to vitamin

TABLE
COMMON FREE RADICALS AND OTHER REACTIVE OXYGEN SPECIES OF BIOLOGICAL IMPORTANCE

| Name | Conventional Symbol | Terminated by Lipoic acid | Terminated by Dihydrolipoic acid |
|---|---|---|---|
| Superoxide anion | $O_2^{\cdot}$ | No | In question, probably not |
| Hydroxyl radical | $HO^{\cdot}$ | Yes | Probably |
| Alkoxyl radical | $RO^{\cdot}$ | ? | ? |
| Peroxyl radical | $ROO^{\cdot}$ | Possibly, but not certain | Possibly, but in doubt |
| Hypochlorous acid | HOCI | Yes | Yes |
| Singlet oxygen | | Yes | Yes (2 of 3 studies) |
| Hydrogen peroxide | $H_2O_2$ | No | No |
| Transition metals | Fe, Cu, Cd, Pb, Hg | Chelates | Chelates |

O = oxygen
H = hydrogen
R = any molecular group
Cl = chlorine
Fe = iron
Cu = copper
Cd = cadmium
Pb = Lead
Hg = mercury

E. And it will reduce the semidehydroascorbyl back to ascorbate (vitamin C). That, in turn, links it to vitamin E, because vitamin C can also reduce the vitamin E radical. So you can see that all these antioxidants are tightly interlinked, with lipoic acid playing a role in recycling many of the key antioxidants in the cell.

When we talk about oxidation and reduction, there are always two compounds involved, one which loses an electron and one which gains an electron. For example, when vitamin E terminates lipid peroxidation, that's an oxidation-reduction reaction. Vitamin E donates an electron to a peroxyl radical. The vitamin E is oxidized and the peroxyl radical is reduced. "Redox" is just a shorthand way of saying "reduction and oxidation," and redox cycles are groups of linked redox reactions. To take the vitamin E example again, after the vitamin E loses an electron, it can be given an electron by another compound, for example, vitamin C. Now the vitamin C has become oxidized, and the vitamin E is reduced—it's been cycled back to its original form.

We discussed how its structure determines lipoic acid's antioxidant capabilities, but let's summarize its actions briefly here.

## LIPOIC ACID—THE IDEAL ANTIOXIDANT

Although there is no one, single perfect antioxidant, lipoic acid is a candidate that approaches that ideal. The antioxidant nutrients are partners working together. Vitamin C, vitamin E and vitamin A are essential vitamins as well as antioxidants. However, they work better when there is more lipoic acid available than what is tied up in use as a coenzyme. Dr. Packer has described an ideal antioxidant as one that has the following biochemical properties:

1. quenches free radicals
2. is easily absorbed and is readily bioavailable
3. concentrates in tissue, cells, and extracellular fluid
4. is present in more than one domain such as aqueous fluids, membranes, cytosol or lipoproteins
5. interacts with other antioxidants
6. chelates free metal ions
7. has positive effects on gene expression

The lipoic acid—dihydrolipoic acid redox couple does all of the above very well.

Lipoic acid can partially replace some of the dietary need for vitamin C and vitamin E. In 1959, Drs. Rosenberg and Culik showed that lipoic acid prevented scurvy in vitamin C-deficient animals, and that it prevented symptoms of vitamin E deficiency in laboratory animals fed a vitamin E-deficient diet. They even predicted that lipoic acid might act as an antioxidant for vitamin C and vitamin E.

Lipoic acid terminates the hydroxyl and hypochlorous free radicals and tests are divided as to whether or not it quenches the peroxyl free radical. Its reduced form, dihydrolipoic acid, also terminates hydroxyl and hypochlorous free radicals, but in addition also terminates superoxide free radicals and definitely quenches peroxyl free radicals. In addition, lipoic acid also quenches the reactive oxygen species singlet oxygen and possibly hydrogen peroxide in some domains but not in others. Results are not yet clear as to whether or not dihydrolipoic acid quenches singlet oxygen.

### LIPOIC ACID INCREASES GLUTATHIONE LEVELS

As part of its regeneration of its partner antioxidant, lipoic acid also increases cellular glutathione content. Glutathione is a major antioxidant within cells. We will discuss this action of lipoic acid further in the sections on cataract and AIDS.

Free radicals are major factors in about 80 diseases, including heart disease, cancer, aging, diabetes, arthritis, cataracts, Alzheimer's disease and many others. Antioxidants destroy free radicals and thus prevent these diseases. Antioxidant nutrients also help alleviate the symptoms and side effects of many of these diseases. Lipoic acid approximates the ideal antioxidant because it is both water- and fat-soluble, works inside and outside of cells, participates in redox cycling, recharges other important antioxidants and quenches several free radicals and reactive oxygen species.

## EFFECT ON GENES AND HEALTH

The excitement soared when it was found that lipoic acid can play a major role in protecting the genes that determine our health. I have been researching antioxidant nutrients since 1959 and I haven't seen this much excitement among researchers since the early days when we learned that free radicals cause many diseases. Now a whole new level of knowledge has been uncovered that explains so much more about why antioxidants in general, and lipoic acid in particular, protect against disease.

Today, we often read that a gene has been found that either causes or increases our susceptibility to develop this or that disease. Therefore, we tend to think that a great deal of disease is genetic in origin. We may rationalize that, since our family is prone to colon cancer or heart disease or whatever, then that's that—if it's all genetic, then why even bother with nutrition and exercise? Well, consider that the gene that causes a particular disease just sits there causing no trouble until hit by a free radical or a certain nuclear factor. Also consider that this gene won't be activated to do its damage if certain antioxidants prevent the free radical or nuclear factor from reaching the gene.

If a particular nuclear factor is activated, it can activate or damage genes, and this in turn determines our health. The discovery of this relationship has only very recently come to light and scientists are very excited as they realize more than ever that antioxidants have great implications for our health.

This section is about the new knowledge that extends our understanding of the role of lipoic acid from just terminating free radicals, but also to protecting the genes from damage from certain nuclear factors. The future may prove that this is the most important part of this chapter, even though it is short.

We can understand the role of lipoic acid with the introduction of just two concepts, genes and a nuclear factor. Free lipoic acid—that is, not tied up as part of the multienzyme complex for energy production—has the ability to protect the genetic material, DNA, in the cell nucleus. A gene is a "block" (segment) of DNA that operates as a unit within a chromosome to control a specific cell function by regulating the production of a specific protein. There are about 100,000 genes in each of the 46 chromosomes in the nucleus of cells. Genes are capable of reproducing themselves at each cell division, and they are capable of managing the formation of body proteins through processes called gene expression and regulation. Any factor that interferes with normal gene regulation can profoundly influence health and lifespan. Free radicals and other reactive oxygen species can influence gene expression and regulation.

Genes can be activated by a protein complex called Nuclear Factor kappa-B (NF-kappa-B).[9] This activator can bind to DNA in genes and cause changes in the rate of gene activation. Old animals, including man, have more NF-kappa-B bound to their genes than do young animals. The most-studied effect of NF-kappa-B has been its effect on the immune system, but it is also known to lead to such things as defective skin cells and aged skin, and apparently can also be responsible for defective cells in all organs, with consequent impaired function of all body systems.

This gene activator, NF-kappa-B, is held in check by other protein sub-units called I-kappa-B proteins. When an I-kappa-B protein binds to NF-kappa-B, the complex cannot pass from the cell cytoplasm through the porous two-layered membrane of the nuclear envelope into the nucleus where the genes are located. The goal for health is not to allow excess NF-kappa-B to be released from the complex, and to permit the body to control its release by normal processes. However, free radicals, peroxides, and ultra-violet energy can induce the inactive complex to dissociate and allow the NF-kappa-B to penetrate into the nucleus and damage DNA.

Antioxidants, by virtue of the fact that they can inhibit free radicals and other reactive oxygen species, are able to inhibit activation of this transcription factor. Lipoic acid is of particular interest because it is where the action is—in the cell interior, the cytosol. An advantage of lipoic acid is that it is a relatively very small molecule and is readily transported through cellular membranes, including the nuclear membrane. It can therefore not only terminate free radicals in the bloodstream and on the cellular membrane, but protect NF-kappa-B in the cytosol and even protect the DNA in the nucleus.

The interaction of the redox couples of lipoic acid/dihydrolipoic acid and glutathione/reduced glutathione on the regulation of NF-kappa-B, tumor necrosis factor and the growth-regulating gene c-fos are complex. Future research will explain more about them and how lipoic acid can help us maintain optimal health.

This section is intended to give you an introduction to the role of lipoic acid and gene expression. Gene expression will be discussed further in the sections on cancer and AIDS. Now that we have covered how lipoic acid protects us against disease by terminating free radicals and protecting our genes, we can look at its role in specific diseases.

## SLOWING AGING

There are many benefits to slowing the aging process besides looking younger longer. A more important benefit is that slowing the rate at which your body ages also delays the occurrence of the so-called age-related diseases. In fact, they can be postponed right out of your lifespan! This section is about how we can achieve the goal of living better longer.

Although the aging process appears very complex when viewed as a group of specific chemical reactions, we can simplify matters by concentrating primarily on the loss of information in the molecules responsible for reproducing the body's proteins. Free radicals and glycation are the responsible culprits. We have already discussed free radicals. Glycation is the modification of a protein by the action of a sugar molecule. Lipoic acid is doubly protective against aging because it protects against free radicals and glycation.

Aging can best be described as the process that reduces the number of healthy cells in the body. Although we have noted the increase of some enzymes in the body, and the decrease of others, the most striking factor in the aging process is the body's loss of reserves needed to respond to a challenge to its status quo (homeostasis).

What causes the body to lose its capacity to respond to a threat? The disappearance of cells from organs and tissues means that there is less of an organ or body system to produce what is needed to counter the threat. The body loses its ability to reproduce some of its cells, and, as cells are destroyed, they are not always replaced.

One by one, the cells disappear until there isn't enough of the working tissue left to handle the challenge.

In addition to the loss of cells, there is a stiffening of tissues. By the mid-1960s it became apparent to me that free radicals could produce cross-linking (which I'll discuss shortly) as well as other damage. Later, I learned that blood sugar could react with body proteins to change their chemical and physical characteristics and cause aging in several ways, primarily by cross-linking and stiffening tissues and organs. Together, the loss of cells and the linking or stiffening of tissues age our bodies.

In 1970, my aging research was sufficiently advanced so that the antioxidant combinations were granted patents in several countries. My main contribution was the concept of the biological synergism of the antioxidant nutrients. The synergism approach made the antioxidant approach practical for humans. Dr. Denham Harman had developed the free-radical theory of aging, but he was working with single nutrients that had to be taken in very large—and impractical—amounts. My unified theory of aging was presented to the 23rd meeting of the Gerontological Society in Toronto on October 21, 1970, and reported in *Chemical & Engineering News* on October 26, 1970.

One major process that accelerates aging occurs when oxygen radicals cause a change in body proteins to produce oxygen-damaged proteins. To lessen damage from radicals, one merely needs to optimize antioxidant nutrient intake. This approach has proved to be very effective against secondary aging effects, and can lead to an additional five to fifteen years of life and disease prevention, depending on when an individual starts the program.

## HOW FREE RADICALS ACCELERATE AGING

The aging of the body through its loss of cells is caused largely by free radical reactions. There are five main ways in which free radicals age the body.

1. Lipid peroxidation, in which free radicals damage fatty compounds,

causing them to essentially turn rancid and to release more free radicals in a chain reaction.

2. Cross-linking, in which free radicals cause proteins and/or DNA to fuse together. DNA is the core of the genetic material that replicates the body components, and altered DNA can't make what the body needs. Instead, useless debris is formed which clogs the body's mechanism and wastes nutrients and other needed factors.
3. Membrane damage, in which free radicals destroy the integrity of cell membranes. This interferes with the cell's ability to absorb nutrients and expel waste products. Both events kill cells.
4. Lysosomal damage, in which free radicals rupture lysosome membranes. Lysosomes are enzymes that can digest just about anything except the membranes that store them. When the membrane sac that stores them is ruptured, the lysosomes spill into the cell interior (cytosol) and destroy critical parts including the nuclei and mitochondria. The cells will then die without being able to reproduce.
5. Miscellaneous free radical reactions form residues called lipofuscin or age pigment. These residues accumulate with time and interfere with cell function and the life process.

All five of these processes destroy vital cells, and with each cell removed from our vital tissues we become one cell older.[12]

## GLYCATION

Blood sugar (glucose) and other sugars called reducing sugars, such as fructose and ribose, react spontaneously—without the need for enzymes—with collagen, a major protein found in skin, blood vessels and connective tissue, and other proteins to form cross-linked sugar-damaged proteins.

The rate of sugar modification of proteins is proportional to sugar concentration. As we discussed earlier, the process of forming these sugar-damaged proteins is called glycation. The actual sugar-damaged proteins and complex derivatives of glucose themselves are called advanced glycosylation end products, AGEs for short. That's not a bad acronym as AGEs lead to a prematurely aged body. AGEs are yellowish-brown fluorescent structures. Glycation can be compared to the browning reaction in toast and sliced apples. The formation rate of AGEs increases as the blood sugar level increases and the length of time the level is raised increases.

The spontaneous reaction of sugar with tissue proteins such as collagen and myelin is responsible for accelerated tissue aging in diabetics, is believed responsible for kidney damage, and is also involved in the atherosclerosis process, which are both common complications of diabetes. Dr. Anthony Cerami observed that glycation reactions also play a role in the normal aging of tissue. This observation led to his glycation hypothesis of aging. Recent studies show that diabetics as well as aging animals do indeed have increased concentrations of AGEs in their collagen. Of related interest is the fact that average blood sugar levels tend to rise with increasing age, owing to the fact that the tissues become less sensitive to the actions of insulin as we age. This reduced sensitivity is not just a loss of reserve due to aging and the loss of tissue, but directly involves the interaction of insulin and the tissues themselves.

The roles of oxygen- and sugar-damaged protein definitely explain much of the secondary aging effects and some of the primary aging process. It appears likely that, other factors being equal, high or widely fluctuating blood sugar levels increase the cross-linking of collagen and other important proteins. Conversely, maintaining precise blood sugar control at the optimal level throughout life should result in tissues that are "young for their age."

## SYNERGISM OF ANTIOXIDANTS AND ANTIGLYCATION

Evidence also suggests that the antioxidant and glycation approaches may be synergistic. Remember, it is not a matter of simply living longer. Both free radical reduction and glycation reduction reduce the incidence of the aging diseases—including heart disease, arthritis and cancer. They are complementary approaches that enhance each other's benefits. Synergy is also involved. As an example, the protection against free-radical damage is more efficient with both approaches than through the actions of either alone.

Studies by Dr. Hans Tritschler at the University of Heidelberg in Germany have shown that the nonenzymatic joining of sugar to protein to form AGEs causes a release of oxygen radicals after binding to receptors.

Some types of cellular damage caused by radicals can be repaired by enzymes. Some enzymes are made solely to repair damage to cells caused by radicals and by high levels of blood sugar.

Antioxidants reduce the damage that radicals do to cell components and the enzymes that repair cells by reducing oxygen modification of proteins. However, without the additional action to prevent the formation of sugar-damaged enzymes, these enzymes will become inactive and unable to repair cell damage. Even though the repair enzymes are protected by antioxidant nutrients, the damage caused by high blood sugar levels quickly becomes significant.

Lipoic acid reduces the protein damage that high blood sugar levels cause. With lipoic acid's antiglycation action to prevent the damage from blood sugar, and its antioxidant action to protect against free radicals, the minor damage that does occur can be repaired by the still-functioning enzymes. The result is that the cell is protected and the body does not become damaged and thereby one cell older.

Lipioc acid reduces glycation and free radical damage. This should prove in the future to have profound practical implications for health and longevity.

The stability of the living system becomes progressively impaired by chemical reactions, not the passage of time. If we can control the rate of these deleterious reactions, we can control the aging process.

## HEART DISEASE PREVENTION AND TREATMENT

Lipoic acid helps prevent heart disease and should be used in its treatment. Through its metabolic role, lipoic acid can lower cholesterol levels by 40 percent, according to laboratory animal studies. In addition, via its antioxidant role, lipoic acid protects against heart disease by its action in the cholesterol carriers called lipoproteins. Research since the 1980s has shown that it is not so important how much cholesterol is in the blood—although that is a factor—but whether or not the carrier of cholesterol has been damaged.

I have been researching heart disease and antioxidant nutrients since 1972. My emphasis has been on vitamin E. Lipoic acid is of interest because it is now known that it plays an important role in maintaining vitamin E in the active form needed to protect against heart disease.

In 1972, I published, "Dietary cholesterol: Is it related to serum cholesterol or heart disease?" in *American Laboratory*. This report established that blood cholesterol was not related to dietary cholesterol in the majority of people, and that dietary cholesterol was poorly related to heart disease. This was heresy in those days.[11]

In 1974, *Prevention* magazine allowed me to conduct a survey of 18,000 of their readers. The study was primarily designed to determine if vitamin E supplementation benefited heart patients. An unexpected finding was that not only did vitamin E benefit actual heart patients, it greatly reduced the incidence of heart disease. The data indicated that length of time that vitamin E was consumed was a more important factor than how much vitamin E was taken. These findings were published in several issues of *Prevention* magazine during 1976, and again in my 1978 book *Supernutrition For Healthy Hearts*.

In May of 1993, two Harvard University School of Medicine studies were published back to back in the *New England Journal of Medicine* showing that vitamin E supplementation over 100 milligrams per day reduced the risk of heart disease by more than 40 percent. (*NEJM* 1993; 328: 1449-56). One, led by Dr. Meir Stampfer, was a study of female nurses, while the other, led by Dr. Eric Rimm, was a study of male health professionals.

## PROTECTING THE CHOLESTEROL CARRIERS

There are several mechanisms that explain why vitamin E directly protects, and lipoic acid indirectly protects, against heart disease. One of these is the protection vitamin E affords the cholesterol carriers called lipoproteins. So let's take a minute or two and discuss lipoproteins. What are they, what do they do and why do we care?

There is no questioning that deposits can form in arteries and reduce the amount of blood that can travel through them and also set the stage for blood clots to form. A heart attack occurs when the heart doesn't get enough blood to provide fuel and oxygen. The formation of a blood clot is called thrombosis. When a clot forms in a narrowed coronary artery, it is called a coronary thrombosis. When the blood clot shuts off the blood supply, the tissue that the artery is supposed to feed will die. When a coronary thrombosis starves a section of the heart (myocardium), this section of tissue will die. The death of tissue is called infarction, so that a heart attack is called a myocardial infarction, sometimes an acute myocardial infarction.

There are thus two main points to address in preventing a heart attack. First, prevent the deposit from forming, and second, prevent the blood from clotting. Vitamin E can do both, and thus offers two-stage protection against heart attacks.

Now let's consider how these deposits form. They are invariably called cholesterol deposits because they contain cholesterol, which makes them visible as white areas.

The deposits depend more on the condition of the cholesterol carriers than on the amount of cholesterol being carried. Cholesterol is a fatty material, and it is not soluble in blood, which is primarily water. Almost everyone knows that oil (fat) is not soluble in water. This is why we use soap to dissolve oil and grime from our hands and clothes. One end of the soap molecules has an affinity for water, while the other end has an affinity for fat. Thus, soap can grab a fatty material and carry it away in water.

This would not work too well in the body. So the body has designed a better transport system for fats in the bloodstream. Proteins have regions that are water-compatible and other regions that are fat-compatible. Our bodies assemble a group of proteins into a hollow ball—actually a sphere-shaped particle. The proteins are aligned in such a way that all the water-friendly ends are on the outside perimeter of the particle, and all the fat-friendly ends are on the inside.

This particle, called a lipoprotein, can now carry fatty compounds in its center, where they will be shielded from the water that is the major component of the blood. The liver packages fatty compounds such as fatty acids, triglycerides and cholesterol into lipoproteins called low-density lipoprotein (LDL) to transport them to the cells where they will be used. Then the liver sends out another carrier, called high-density lipoprotein, to retrieve any excess fatty materials not used. Cells can build receptors that grab either LDL or HDL as needed. The system is apparently perfect, cholesterol transport is under strict control, both to and from the cells.

However, LDL can become damaged by oxidation or free radicals due to insufficient antioxidant levels. Such damaged LDL is called oxidized-LDL (Ox-LDL). Ox-LDL is taken up by scavenger receptors in artery cells. A long process is triggered, which need not be discussed here, but the essence is that when Ox-LDL enters artery cells, the immune system sends monocytes to attempt to rid the cells of the damaged LDL. Some of these monocytes are converted into macrophages. Both macrophages and monocytes are white blood cells. Their appearance in the cells is called foam cell formation because this is what the lipid-laden white cells look like—foam in the artery cells. When more Ox-LDL enters the artery cells than can be handled by the monocytes, the cells become damaged and deposits build up. This discussion, of course, is an oversimplification, but it serves to illustrate that the big culprit in heart disease is inadequate antioxidants, not too much cholesterol. The cholesterol in normal LDL and HDL is not a factor in forming the deposits. It is primarily the cholesterol in the Ox-LDL that forms the deposits.

LDL cholesterol is often called the bad cholesterol while HDL cholesterol is called the good cholesterol. However, LDL cholesterol is "bad" only when it has been oxidized. The cholesterol carried in

LDL, HDL, and Ox-LDL is cholesterol. Cholesterol is cholesterol is cholesterol! It is only the condition of the lipoprotein particle that is carrying it that makes the difference.

Now what does all of this have to do with lipoic acid? The lipoproteins carry the fat-soluble antioxidant nutrients as well as the fatty materials. The fat-soluble antioxidants are carried along with the fats to protect them from oxidation. If we are well-nourished, our LDL doesn't become damaged. Vitamin E is the primary protector of LDL. However, vitamin E could quickly be consumed by free radicals if it didn't have antioxidant partners to protect it or recycle it back to its undamaged form, tocopherol.

Here's where lipoic acid comes in. Lipoic acid is transported in LDL with vitamin E. As we discussed earlier, lipoic acid can directly and indirectly recharge vitamin E so that it can keep on protecting LDL. In addition, lipoic acid directly protects LDL itself. This, lipoic acid offers double-barreled protection of LDL.

## LIPOIC ACID IN THE TREATMENT OF HEART DISEASE

Several researchers in the former U.S.S.R. have shown that lipoic acid lowers cholesterol in animals, notably Dr. V. E. Anisimov in 1969 and Dr. S. A. Koziov in 1971. The research that I report here is by Dr. V. N. Ivanov of the Department of Biochemistry of the Medical Institute of Chita in the former U.S.S.R. in 1974. Dr. Ivanov noted that since lipoic acid favorably influences the metabolism of carbohydrates, proteins and fats, which are disturbed in heart patients, lipoic acid might be of value in lowering blood cholesterol. In 1960, Dr. C. Dojama found that lipoic acid was an antiatherogenic agent as it activated the oxioreductive enzymes involved in fat breakdown.

Dr. Ivanov used rabbits for his studies, because they were used for most of the prior cholesterol studies done around the world. He found that lipoic acid reduced total blood cholesterol by 40 percent and cholesterol in aortic tissue by 45 percent. He also reported that lipoic acid reduced blood LDL levels by 42 percent and aortic LDL levels by 45 percent.

The net result of Dr. Ivanov's experiments was that lipoic acid improved the amount of oxygen actually getting to the heart. Lipoic acid enhanced oxygen uptake in the heart by 72 percent, by 148 percent in the aorta, and by 128 percent in the liver.

Dr. Ivanov concluded, "The results achieved justify a recommendation of lipoic acid for wide usage in the treatment of patients with atherosclerosis."

Lipoic acid protects against heart disease both via its metabolic role and via its antioxidant role. The dual roles of lipoic acid, the metabolic antioxidant, once again offer complete modes of protection. The results of Dr. C. Ivanov justify using lipoic acid in the treatment of heart disease.

## CANCER

Today, it is fairly common knowledge that antioxidant nutrients protect against some cancers. The evidence began with laboratory animal studies decades ago and has been supported by epidemiological (population) studies. At this writing several clinical intervention studies are under way. When all of the evidence is in, perhaps by the year 2010 or so, we will have fairly definitive proof. What we have today is an appreciable body of evidence that unquestionably demonstrates that those who eat diets rich in fruits and vegetables are at lower risk to develop cancer. We also have reasonable evidence from animal, mechanistic and epidemiological studies that the protective factors in fruits and vegetables are primarily antioxidant nutrients including vitamin C, vitamin E, carotenoids, bioflavonoids and other antioxidant nutrients. While we wait for the final results, it is prudent to make sure that we get optimal amounts of the various antioxidant nutrients, including lipoic acid, which spares and regenerates its other antioxidant partners.

In this section, we will discuss how antioxidant nutrients in general protect against cancer, and how lipoic acid also protects the nuclear factor that prevents oncogene activation.

When I examined the incidence of cancer in my laboratory animals in my aging experiments, I did confirm a drastically lower incidence rate. I then conducted a series of experiments to study the possibility that the synergistic antioxidants were protective against cancer. They were.

In 1972, I filed for international patent protection for various combinations of nutrients that protected against cancer. I published my first results in *American Laboratory* in 1973 and have been issued patents on antioxidant synergism in the prevention of cancer. I continued my research and published *Supernutrition: Megavitamin Therapy* in 1975 and *Cancer and Its Nutritional Therapies* in 1978. This was updated as *Cancer Prevention and Nutritional Therapies* in 1993.[15]

Even in the 1978 edition, I cited hundreds of studies that showed that the deficiencies of certain antioxidant nutrients increased the occurrence of both spontaneous and induced cancers. Conversely, many studies showed a dose-dependent relationship to lowered incidence of many cancers. That is, the more of the antioxidant nutrients consumed, the greater the reduction in cancer rates. This, too, was shown for spontaneous and induced cancers.

## WHAT IS CANCER?

Cancer is actually a group of diseases. There are 100 different types of cancers. What they have in common is that each is a disease of the body's cells. Most cancers involve tumors. Healthy cells grow, divide and replace themselves in an orderly way. A mutation can make cells lose their ability to limit and direct their growth. They divide too rapidly and grow without order. Too much tissue is produced and tumors are formed. Tumors can be benign or malignant. Malignant tumors are cancers, and they can spread and invade other parts of the body.

## HOW LIPOIC ACID PROTECTS AGAINST CANCER

Lipoic acid can help keep cells from going astray. Earlier, we discussed how lipoic acid protected a complex called Nuclear Factor kappa-B, and prevented it from activating oncogenes. Oncogenes are genes that cause cancer. Oncogenes normally play a role in the growth and proliferation of cells, but when they are altered in some way such as by the activated NF-kappa-B or a carcinogen, they cause the cell to become malignant. Dietary lipoic acid can enter the cytosol of cells and protect NF-kappa-B from activation by radiation, free radicals or even sunlight.

We discussed earlier how antioxidants terminate free radicals. Free radicals can damage the sensors on cell membranes that signal the cell when to divide for growth. If the sensors are damaged, then unregulated growth can occur. Unregulated cell growth is the operative word in cancer.[15]

If a free radical reacts with DNA in the nucleus, then the gene may produce an incorrect protein and the cell becomes altered or mutated. Free radicals can also impair the immune system, which would otherwise recognize and destroy mutated cells before they multiply and become cancer.

Since lipoic acid is a small molecule that is both water-soluble and fat-soluble, it can enter all body domains and terminate free radicals before they have a chance to cause the damage that can lead to cancer.

Lipoic acid protects against cancer by protecting NF-kappa-B from being activated to genes, and by its nearly universal presence as a powerful antioxidant to prevent membrane and DNA damage.[16,17]

## DIABETES

Lipoic acid is a very important nutrient for diabetics—it would not be an exaggeration to call it a blessing. Lipoic acid not only normalizes blood sugar levels in diabetics, it protects against the damage responsible for diabetes in the first place. It has been successfully used in Germany for more than 30 years, where it has reduced the secondary effects of diabetes, including damage to the retina, cataract formation, nerve and heart damage, as well as increasing energy levels.[18, 19, 20]

Diabetes strikes one of every twenty Americans. Not only is it the third leading cause of death in the U.S., it inflicts serious suffering in the form of blindness, nerve damage, heart disease, gangrene, and amputated limbs. In little more than a generation, the incidence of diabetes has increased over 600 percent, accounting for 300,000 to 350,000 deaths each year during the early 1990s. About half of those with coronary artery disease and three-fourths of those suffering strokes develop their circulatory problems prematurely as a result of diabetes.

Diabetes is a group of diseases in which the body cannot properly metabolize food into energy. The result is a build-up of blood sugar that causes the long-term glycation damage we discussed earlier, and is responsible for even more immediate problems. The high sugar level in the blood results in osmotic changes and reduced blood volume, shock, acidosis, coma and death. Insulin-dependent diabetes mellitus (type I) normally results when the body does not produce enough insulin.[21] This is normally the result of damage to the beta cells of the pancreas. This form of diabetes usually, but not always, begins in childhood and was often called juvenile diabetes.[22, 23, 24]

Non-insulin dependent diabetes (type II) accounts for about 85 percent of diabetes cases and is usually associated with age and/or obesity. It is still sometimes called adult-onset diabetes. This form of diabetes is caused by insulin resistance of peripheral cells or the inability of insulin receptors to utilize insulin efficiently. Usually, diet and oral medication can keep blood sugar levels near normal, but insulin is generally of no value. Type II diabetics generally have high levels of insulin in the blood, but it is ineffective because of the insulin resistance of the tissues.

Unhappily, even when blood sugar levels are reduced below a critical level, they still fluctuate widely and are still above the level that leads to glycation. Glycation damage and free radical damage lead to such diabetic complications as cataract, retinopathy, stiffened arteries and heart tissue, damaged lipoproteins (Ox-LDL) and nerve destruction.

Lipoic acid can terminate free radicals and thus reduce the oxidative stress that can damage the pancreas, cause cataracts, nerve damage, retinopathy and other side effects. Lipoic acid also reduces glycation, which otherwise can damage proteins, especially those of skin and blood vessels. Even more important to diabetics is that lipoic acid, by virtue of its ability to normalize blood sugar level and the entire glycolysis pathway for conversion of sugar into energy, allows the nerves to recover. Pain is reduced and normal feeling is restored.

Lipoic acid acts to increase glucose transport by stimulating the glucose transporters (a type of protein) GLUT-1 and GLUT-4 to move from the cell interior to the membrane.[25, 26] This action is independent of insulin transport. It is believed that the sulfur atoms of lipoic acid are responsible for the translocation action. This restoration of normal blood sugar level in turn increases the number of glucose transporters in the membranes of muscle cells. This is a very desirable cycle.

Lipoic acid supplementation at the level of 300 to 600 milligrams per day has been efficient in significantly lowering blood sugar, sorbitol, serum pyruvate and acetoacetate levels while increasing glycogen (stored energy compound for muscles) in muscles and the liver. At the same time, there is an increase in blood sugar utilization by muscle tissues and a reduction in liver glucose output.

## IMPROVED NEUROLOGICAL FUNCTION

German studies with high doses of lipoic acid in diabetics have shown that it improves peroneal (leg) nerve conduction velocity, as well as heart and gastrointestinal functions.[13]

Dr. D. Ziegler and colleagues at the Heinrich-Heine University in Dusseldorf, Germany have shown that long-term treatment with lipoic acid induces what is known as "sprouting," i.e., the growth of new nerve fibers in a regeneration process. In as little as three weeks there is a significant reduction in pain and numbness. The researchers observed no adverse effects from the high dosage (600 milligrams per day) of lipoic acid.

A review of the literature shows that in cell cultures, lipoic acid causes a dose-dependent sprouting of neurites in nerve cells. This has been attributed to improvement in nerve cell membrane fluidity. In animal experiments, lipoic acid promoted regeneration after partial denervation. Lipoic acid improves the blood flow in nerve tissues, improves glucose utilization in the brain and improves basal ganglia function.

In March, 1995, at an international meeting on diabetic neuropathy, in Munich, Germany, several researchers reported the results of clinical studies in which lipoic acid reversed the damage of diabetes to the nerves, heart and eyes of diabetics.

Most of the clinical studies were from European universities and clinics. Study after study reported that lipoic acid safely regenerated damaged nerves. The consensus was that lipoic acid protects through its antioxidant and antiglycemic actions. The conference concluded that lipoic acid was the agent of choice for the prevention of diabetic complications, including neuropathy, cardiomyopathy and retinopathy.[27]

## INCREASED MUSCLE ENERGY, DECREASED FAT PRODUCTION

At the Munich meeting Dr. Hans Tritschler's group reported additional information on how lipoic acid increases glucose uptake by muscle cells and decreases glucose uptake by fat cells. Dr. M. Khamaisi's group at the University of Negev in Israel reported that the increased glucose transport actually leads to increased energy production. This was confirmed with another study by Dr. Tritschler's group, using phosphorus magnetic resonance spectroscopic studies to show increased metabolism and ATP production in muscle tissues, and improved muscle recovery, which permits more work or exercise to be done.[28, 29]

The result is more energy production in muscles and less fat stored in the body. This is of course of special importance to diabetics who don't wish to, or can't, improve their lifestyle by exercising—but it is also obviously of great interest to everyone else!

## CAUTION

Diabetics may require insulin or oral antidiabetic dose reduction to prevent hypoglycemic states. Close monitoring of blood glucose level is required.

There is absolutely no doubt that all diabetics should be supplementing their diets with lipoic acid! It can mean all the difference in the world. They should also consider supplementation with chromium picolinate. It is imperative that diabetics monitor their blood sugar levels closely and have appropriate adjustments made to their medication doses to prevent lowering their blood sugar levels too far.

## ADDITIONAL PROTECTION

Lipoic acid is important for many more reasons than can be included in this chapter. However, the role of lipoic acid in detoxification, cataract prevention, nerve regeneration, and the immune system enhancement that may prevent HIV infection from developing into clinical AIDS must be mentioned.

### DETOXIFICATION

It is apparent that lipoic acid is itself a versatile and direct antioxidant. However, there is still more to its antioxidant protective actions. It also has an indirect action via its ability to chelate many metals (minerals). To chelate means that a compound can grab a metal atom with "claws" formed by certain groups of atoms in the compound.

Iron and copper are essential nutrients, but excesses or 'free" unbound atoms or ions can be harmful. If iron and copper are present in excess as free, unbound ions, they can be oxidants. Any compound that would chelate free ions of iron and copper would thus indirectly reduce oxidation and be considered an antioxidant. Lipoic acid does not chelate the desirable form of iron that is part of proteins such as hemoglobin or the enzyme catalase, but it appears to be capable of removing iron from the storage protein ferritin in both the ferrous and ferric states. I have not seen studies that would indicate whether lipoic acid would be of value to people with iron overload disorders, but there does seem to be some potential.

In most cases, iron and copper are complexed in the body with other proteins, so the concentration of free metal ions is quite low, but under some conditions of trauma, these metal ions can be released. When that happens, the ability to complex is very important, because that inhibits these ions' catalyzing oxidative processes.

Cadmium, lead and mercury are toxic metals at essentially all levels. Cadmium is a toxic metal that is present in tobacco smoke and accumulates in smokers. It is believed to be responsible for a significant amount of the harm caused by smoking. Lead is a toxic metal that gets into the air we breathe from automobile exhaust. It is also present in many water supplies and processed foods. Mercury is a toxic material present in dental fillings and in fish from mercury-polluted waters.

## CATARACTS

As we age, we are all at risk to develop cataracts, a degeneration of the eye lens. Diabetics are especially at risk, as they have increased oxidative and glycation damage. Excess exposure to sunlight is also a risk factor in the development of cataracts. The ultraviolet energy of sunlight creates free radicals in the tissues it impinges upon. The eye lens is directly exposed to sunlight, and, unfortunately, cells in eye lenses are not directly bathed by antioxidant-rich blood.

It is therefore difficult to keep these lens cells optimally nourished with antioxidant nutrients. Epidemiological studies have confirmed that persons with higher dietary intakes of antioxidant nutrients have a lower incidence of cataracts.

Lipoic acid is not only a powerful antioxidant that can get into cells easily due to its small molecular size and water and fat compatibility, it also facilitates glutathione production in cells. Glutathione is a major cellular antioxidant. Cataract tissues have low glutathione levels. In laboratory animal experiments, Dr. Lester Packer's group has shown that lipoic acid increased levels of glutathione, vitamin C and vitamin E in eye lens tissue (Free Rad. Biol. Med. 1994). Also, cell culture studies have shown that lipoic acid blocks cataract formation in lenses from diabetic rats.

## AIDS

During HIV infection, key cells of the immune system called CD lymphocytes lose their ability to make and to transport glutathione. Since glutathione is a major cellular antioxidant, these immune cells succumb to oxidative stress and the immune system fails. As the immune system becomes impaired, the HIV-positive person increasingly develops opportunistic infections that ordinarily do not infect healthy people, and enters further into clinical AIDS.

This decline may be prevented if the immune cells can keep their antioxidant status sufficiently high. Since lipoic acid is a powerful antioxidant and a facilitator of glutathione production, researchers conducted a small clinical trial that produced such exciting results, other larger studies are being planned at this writing.

Dr. J. Fuchs and colleagues gave 150 milligrams of lipoic acid three times daily for a two-week period and found that plasma glutathione levels increased in all patients, the number of T-helper cells increased in two-thirds of the patients, and the T-helper/T-suppressor cell ratio improved in 60 percent of the patients. (Arzneimittel-Forschung 43:1359-62;1993).

A cell culture study found that lipoic acid prevented the replication of the HIV virus. The HIV virus replicates when NF-kappa-B is activated. We discussed earlier how lipoic acid protects NF-kappa-B from being activated which in turn causes genes to be expressed (to produce more of what it is supposed to produce).

## NEURODEGENERATIVE DISEASES

**Nerve regeneration, Parkinson's disease and Alzheimer's disease.** In the section on diabetes, I discussed how lipoic acid improves nerve transmission and even regenerates nerves in diabetics. The effect of high blood sugar levels is to destroy nerves. The role of lipoic acid is more than just to allow the nerves to regenerate because it lowers blood sugar to normal in diabetics. It also improves membrane fluidity in nondiabetics. We have glycation aging us even if we don't have diabetes. Sugar-damaged proteins are just as harmful as oxygen-damaged proteins. Lipoic acid is protective against both glycation and oxidation. There is even more to the story to learn.

The central nervous system is especially vulnerable to oxidative damage because of its high oxygen consumption. The increased oxygen radical production increases mitochondrial dysfunction, which in turn increases radical production. This leads to cell death in brain and CNS tissue. In neurodegenerative diseases such as Parkinson's disease and Alzheimer's disease, mitochondrial dysfunction and oxidative stress may cause or worsen the clinical features. (Tritschler, H. J.; Packer, L. and Medori, R., Biochem. Mol. Biol. Int. 34:169-81;1994)

Lipoic acid is especially suited to protect nerve tissues against oxidative damage, and has been found to be neuroprotective. (Greenamyre, J. T.; et al., Neurosci. Letters 171:17-20;1994)

In animal studies, 100 milligrams of lipoic acid per kilogram of body weight improved memory even to the point better than that of young animals not given extra lipoic acid. (Stoll, S.; et al., Pharmacol. Biochem. Behav. 46:799-85;1993)

## SAFETY

The miracles of lipoic acid would be of little value unless its use were safe. It is not a matter of more benefit than risk; it is a matter of *primum non nocere:* First, do no harm.

Lipoic acid is made in the body and it is present in the diet. Food tables do not yet include the lipoic acid content of foods. Since lipoic acid is used in mitochondria, foods that are rich in mitochondria are good sources of lipoic acid. The most common foods rich in mitochondria would be red meats because they are some of the richest mitochondria sources. However, today people are deemphasizing red meat in their diets. Another good source of lipoic acid is yeast, which is not a staple of a typical American diet. Fortunately, lipoic acid supplements are available that are not derived from meat or animal products.

No clinical, toxicological or postmarketing studies have shown a serious adverse effect from lipoic acid supplementation, and it has been used for more than three decades at high dosage (300 to 600 milligrams per day) to treat diabetic neuropathy. However, as mentioned in the section on diabetes, diabetics will have improved glucose utilization and should monitor their blood sugar level closely and/or use it with the guidance of their physician.

Studies have not indicated any carcinogenic (cancer-causing) or teratogenic (birth defect) effects. However, as a precaution, until further information is available, lipoic acid supplements are not recommended for pregnant women.

Alcoholics or others who are severely deficient in thiamine (vitamin B1) should be sure to take thiamine supplements along with lipoic acid supplements.

As with any food, there may be a few individuals who will have allergic-type responses such as skin reactions or upset stomach.

The acute toxic dose, expressed as LD50, is 400 to 500 milligrams per kilogram of body weight in several species. This is equivalent to 30,000 to 37,500 milligrams (30 to 37.5 grams) for a 165-pound human.

The typical prophylactic daily supplementation range for healthy adults appears to be 20 to 50 milligrams. Higher amounts may be recommended by health care providers according to the individual needs of their patients.

## REFERENCES

1. Packer, L., Witt, E. H. and Tritschler, H. J. Alpha-lipoic acid as a biological antioxidant. *Free Radical Biol. & Med.* 19(2):227-50, 1995.
2. Passwater, Richard A. Lipoic acid basics. *Whole Foods,* January 1996.
3. Snell, E. E., Tatum, E. L. and Peterson, W. H. *J. Bact.* 33:207, 1937.
4. Guirard, B. M., Snell, E. E. and Williams, R. J. *Arch. Biochem.* 9:381, 1946.
5. Reed, L. J., DeBusk, B. G., Gunsalus, I. C. and Hornberger, Jr., C. S. Crystalline alphalipoic acid: A catalytic agent associated with pyruvate dehydrogenase. *Science* 114(2952):03-4, 1951.
6. Reed, L. J. Multienzyme complexes. *Accounts Chem. Res.* 7:40-46, 1974.

7. Bast, A. and Haenen, G. Interplay between dihydrolipoic acid and glutathione in the protection against microsome lipid peroxidation. *Biochem. Biophys. Acta* 963:558-61, 1988.
8. Kagan, V., et al. Antioxidant action of thioctic acid and dihydrolipoic acid. *Free Rad. Biol. Med.* 95:15, 1990.
9. Shreck, R. et al. Reactive oxygen intermediates as apparently widely used messengers in the activation of NF-kappa-alpha. *EMBO J.* 10:2247-58, 1991.
10. Passwater, Richard A. Plans for a large-scale study of possible retardation of the human aging process. *The Gerontologist* 10(3):11, 28, 1970.
11. Passwater, Richard A. and Welker, P. A. Human Aging Research, Part II. *American Laboratory* 3(5):21-27, 1971.
12. Harman, Denham J. The free-radical theory of aging. *J. Gerontol.* 11:298-300, 1956.
13. Passwater, Richard A. *The Longevity Factor: Chromium Picolinate.* Keats Publishing, Inc., New Canaan, Conn., 1993.
14. Passwater, Richard A. *The New Supernutrition.* Pocket Books, New York, 1991.
15. Passwater, Richard A. *Cancer Prevention and Nutritional Therapies.* Keats Publishing, Inc., New Canaan, Conn. 1993.
16. Krontiris, T. G. Molecular Medicine: Oncogenes. *New Engl. J. Med.* 333(5):303-6, Aug. 3, 1995.
17. Cavenee, W. K. and White, R. L. The genetic basis of cancer. *Sci. Amer.* 72-9, March 1995.
18. Natraj, C. V.; Gandhi, V. M. and Menon, K. K. G. Lipoic acid and diabetes. *J. Biosci.* 6:37-46, 1984.
19. Gandhi, V. M.; Wagh, S. S.; *et al.* Lipoic acid and diabetes II. *J. Biosci.* 9:117-27, 1985. Wagh, S. S.; Gandhi, V. M.; et al. Lipoic acid and diabetes III. *J. Bosci.* 10:171-9, 1986.
20. Wagh, S. S., Natraj, C. V. and Menon, K. K. G. Mode of action of lipoic acid in diabetes III. *J. Biosci.* 11:59-74, 1987.
21. Faust, A., Burkart, V.; *et al.* Effect of lipoic acid and insulitis in non-obese diabetic mice. *Int. J. Immunopharmac* 16:61-66, 1994.
22. Burkart, V., Koike, T., *et al.* Dihydrolipoic acid protects pancreatic islet cells. *Agents and Actions* 38:60-5, 1993.
23. Haugaard, N. and Haugaard, E. S. Stimulation of glucose utilization by thioctic acid. *Biophys. Acta* 222:583-6, 1970.
24. Singh, H. P. P. and Bowman R. H. Effect of lipoic acid. *Biochem. Biophys. Res. Com.* 41:555-61, 1970.

25. Bashan, N.; Burdett, E.; *et al.* Effect of thiotic acid on glucose transport. In: Gries, F. A. and Wessel, K., eds. *The role of antioxidants in diabetes mellitus.* PMI-Verlag-Gruppe;1993:221-9.
26. Henriksen, E. J.; Jacob, S.; Tritschler, H.; *et al.* Chronic thiotic acid treatment increases insulin-stimulated glucose transport activity. *Diabetes. Suppl.* 1:122A abstract; 1994.
27. Sachse, G. and Willms, B. Horm. Efficiency of thioctic acid in the therapy of peripheral diabetic neuropathy. *Metab. Res. Supp.* Ser 9:105, 1980.
28. Klip, A.; Volchuk, A.; Ramlal, T.; *et al.* Glucose transporters of muscle cells in culture. In: Draznin, B. and LeRoith, D., eds. *Molecular Biology of Diabetes.* Humana Press, Totowa, N.J., 1994.
29. Reschke, B.; Zeuzem, S.; Rosak, C.; *et al.* High-dose long-term treatment with thioctic acid in diabetic polyneuropathy. In: Borbe/Ulrich, eds., *Thioctsaure:* 318-34, 1989.

# PART FOUR

# FATS IN HEALTH AND DISEASE

# INTRODUCTION

MOST OF US have been trained since early childhood to associate dietary fat with negative images: being overweight or obese, as being sinful (as in "everything I like is immoral, illegal or fattening"), and being unhealthy—contributing to heart disease, diabetes and cancer. Even the word itself is often used in a derogatory way: "Hey, fathead" or "Fat chance you have" or "Let's trim the fat"—no one says "Fat as a fiddle."

## ALL FATS ARE NOT CREATED EQUAL

As you have learned from this book, fats can be harmful or beneficial, depending on chemical structure. We know we must eat foods containing the essential fatty acids such as the omega-3 and omega-6 forms because they have important, life-supporting roles in human nutrition. They are essential to infants and children for proper growth, necessary to prevent drying and flaking skin, are an integral part of cell membranes, regulators of cholesterol metabolism and provide the raw material for hormone-like substances such as prostaglandins. Prostaglandins help regulate many processes in the body: inflammation, healing and repair, immunity, neural circuits in the brain, the cardiovascular, digestive and reproductive systems, and your body thermostat. It is obvious that imbalances or deficiencies in these fats can cause many problems.

## IT TAKES FAT TO LOSE FAT

Fats can also be ideal diet aids. They are satisfying and filling and can actually reduce the craving for food, so even dieters need to get at least 25 percent of their calories from fat. Fat in the stomach slows digestion time, so that you are not hungry "five minutes later." By slowing digestion and allowing proteins to be fully digested, fats may also decrease allergic food reactions. Undigested proteins often cause stronger allergies.

Fats are also necessary for the absorption of key vitamins—A, D, E and K—from the diet. A very low-fat diet will result in deficiencies of these nutrients, and make dieting more difficult. If you are already low in key nutrients, and then go on a diet which further reduces these nutrients, you will not have the stamina or health to stick to the diet. Essential fatty acids are actually fats that help you lose weight. Unlike the saturated and trans fats, the good fats increase the metabolic rate and the efficiency of processes that burn fat. Strict dieting decreases the metabolic rate making it more difficult to lose fat.

## BY LAND OR BY SEA

There are many beneficial effects of essential fatty acids in health and especially in disease states. Whether from land or from the sea, these good fats and oils improve the quality of life. The best sources of omega-3s are fatty fish like salmon, mackerel, sardines, herring, anchovies, whitefish and bluefish. Swordfish, rainbow trout, striped bass, Pacific oysters and squid contain fair amounts as well. But there are other non-fish sources. Linolenic acid, a fatty acid found in some plants, can be converted by the body to eicosapentaenoic acid (EPA) and docosahexaenoic acid (DHA), the essential omega-3s found in fish oil. Plant sources of linolenic acid include linseed oils, walnuts and walnut oil, flaxseed, rapeseed (used to make canola oil), soybeans, spinach, mustard greens and purslane.

## A FISHY STORY

During the 1980s, many researchers reported that omega-3 fatty acids helped protect against the ravages of heart disease, cancer and inflammatory diseases like rheumatoid arthritis. Newspapers and magazines carried pictures of healthy Eskimos and everyone ran for the sardines. But then, as with all "new" nutritional therapies, contradictory evidence led to confusion and then indifference.

Well, we all owe Grandma (or Mom) an apology. We need to say "sorry" for every face we made when she made us swallow that big spoonful of cod liver oil. Although she may not have had a medical degree, she knew—from experience and folklore—that fish oil was good for you. Just how good is becoming more and more evident to scientists and researchers alike.

### CLEAR EVIDENCE—THE FISH DID IT

As the research continued, omega-3 fatty acids came back in favor. In the spring of 1993, the American Heart Association held a world-wide conference to discuss the latest findings on the role of omega-3s in human health and how that information translated into dietary recommendations.

A string of positive findings was confirmed at the conference by such noted researchers as William Connor M.D. of the University of Iowa and Alexander Leaf M.D., of Harvard Medical School. Omega-3s lower blood pressure, reduce serum triglyceride levels and increase clotting times thus decreasing the risk of cardiovascular disease and stroke. Omega-3s also slow or prevent cancerous tumor growth, especially in colon cancer. Ulcerative colitis and lung disease benefit from fish or fish oil supplementation of the diet. Fish oils prevent blood vessels from closing following vascular surgery, improve inflammatory diseases like rheumatoid arthritis and relieve symptoms of psoriasis.

## FATS AND DISEASE

### RHEUMATOID ARTHRITIS

In populations with high intakes of omega-3 fatty acids, chronic inflammatory diseases such as rheumatoid arthritis appear to be less common or milder than in groups following conventional Western diets. In a Danish study, patients taking fish oil capsules (containing a total of 3.6 grams per day of omega-3 fatty acids) reported significant improvement of morning stiffness and joint tenderness.

In the European *Journal of Clinical Investigations* in 1992, G. L.

Nielsen and colleagues in Denmark reported that dietary supplementation with omega-3 fatty acid containing fish oil resulted in improvement in patients with rheumatoid arthritis.

Fish or fish oil should become a regular part of the diet. "It may take three to four months to see the benefits from a diet that regularly includes fish," says Joel M. Kremer, M.D., head of the division of rheumatology at Albany Medical College.

## CARDIOVASCULAR DISEASE

The omega-3 fatty acids are thought to reduce the risk of heart disease by lowering blood cholesterol and reducing blood clot formation. Researchers followed 44,895 healthy men with no heart disease who gave detailed information on their eating habits for ten years. Men who ate fish had a lower risk of developing fatal heart disease than those who did not. Whether they ate fish six times a week, or once a week on average, the risk of heart disease was the same.

Writing in the *American Journal of Clinical Nutrition* in 1992, Kaj N. Seidelin and colleagues in Denmark reported that, in 40 consecutive autopsies, the highest degree of coronary artery disease was associated with lower concentrations of the essential oil DHA.

Isabelle Bairati M.D., Ph.D. and colleagues reported in the *Canadian Journal of Cardiology,* in 1992, that fish oil supplementation had a beneficial effect on blood pressure and serum triglycerides in patients treated for coronary artery disease and who had high blood pressure. In another study, it was shown that regular intake of fish oil reduces triglyceride levels after eating.

In a 15-year study of 552 men, Dutch researchers found that those who ate a serving of fish every day (20 grams) had almost half the risk of stroke compared with men who ate less. The effect may be due to a reduction in platelet aggregation, as reported in the journal *Stroke* (1994;25:328-332).

Between 30 and 45 percent of patients who undergo coronary angioplasty, a procedure to widen clogged blood vessels, develop restenosis (re-blockage) within six months after treatment. There is no known medical therapy to prevent restenosis, but researchers from the Medical College of Wisconsin analyzed a number of studies to determine the possible therapeutic effects of fish oils. The researchers stated that the analysis supported the hypothesis that fish oil, containing the omega-3 fatty acids, was effective in reducing restenosis following angioplasty.

## COLON CANCER

In animal experiments, the two major omega-3 fatty acids in fish oils, EPA and DHA, inhibit both the initiation and promotion phases of the development of colon tumors. Epidemiologic studies have also linked high consumption of fish products with a low rate of colorectal cancer. At the Catholic University of Rome, the effect of omega-3 fatty acids on colorectal cancer risk was investigated in high risk patients with a history of colorectal polyps. There was significant decrease in cells considered reliable markers of colon cancer risk after two weeks of treatment.

Fish oil supplements were also shown to reduce the proliferation of rectal cells in a study by Dr. Hans-Peter Bartram published in *Gastroenterology* (1993;105:1317-1322). There was also a reduction in the activity of an enzyme, ornithine decarboxylase. Increased activity of this enzyme has been documented in patients with familial colonic polyposis, a condition that increases the risk of colon cancer. The findings support the idea that fish in the diet is at least in part responsible for the low colon cancer rates in Alaskan and Greenland Eskimos.

## ULCERATIVE COLITIS

For people struggling with ulcerative colitis, fish oil may help control their diarrhea, cramping and gas pains, according to a study in the American *Journal of Gastroenterology*, April 1992. No one with ulcerative colitis, however, should start taking fish oil without talking it over with their doctor first.

## SMOKERS GO FISH

Smokers who eat plenty of fish may lower their risk of chronic lung disease, a major hazard of cigarettes, according to a study of 8,960 current and former smokers published in the July 28, 1994 issue of the *New England Journal of Medicine.* Dr. Eyal Shahar, the lead researcher of the study done at the University of Minnesota, Minneapolis, found that frequent fish eaters were significantly less likely to suffer emphysema (two-thirds lower risk) and bronchitis (one-third lower risk) than smokers who ate less fish. Experts believe that smoking causes lung disease by triggering inflammation in the lungs and that fish oil (containing EPA and DHA) may protect by inhibiting this response. Emphysema and bronchitis result in 75,000 deaths in the United States each year.

## FISH SKIN

In his book, *Natural Prescriptions,* Robert M. Giller, M.D., stated that fish oil applied to the skin, gives relief to patients with psoriasis. There is a great deal of evidence that fish oils also protect and "lubricate" the joints, aiding in relief from arthritis, according to Dr. Giller. The best natural sources are herring, salmon, bluefish and tuna. Fish oil supplements found in health food stores are also beneficial in relieving the symptoms of arthritis, he added.

## DIABETES

Fish oils containing omega-3 fatty acids have been shown to be beneficial in reducing the risk of cardiovascular disease. This might seem to be welcome news for diabetics, who are at particularly high risk for cardiovascular disease. However, fish oil has caused problems with sugar control and blood fat levels in diabetics. The studies that found these effects occurred, however, when researchers used high (and possibly excessive) doses of fish oil.

In a study conducted at Massachusetts General Hospital, using a lower dose of fish oil such as that found in a fish-rich diet, patients receiving fish oil showed a significant decrease in platelet aggregation, decreasing the risk of blood clots. They also showed a reduction in triglyceride levels. Fish oil caused small but significant increases in glycated hemoglobin (a measure of sugar control) and total cholesterol, but the authors concluded that low doses of fish oil were safe for diabetics. They indicated that beneficial effects on platelet aggregation probably outweighed the small undesirable changes and that fish was a good replacement for red meat, which is high in undesirable saturated fatty acids.

## MORE OIL BENEFITS

Patients with kidney transplants who took fish oil for one year had a lower incidence of acute rejection episodes, according to a study published in the *New England Journal of Medicine* (1993;329:769-773).

Mastodynia, pain in the breast, can be effectively treated with evening primrose oil. Evening primrose oil is also used to treat premenstrual syndrome (PMS).

## DON'T FORGET THE FLAX

Plant sources supply one type of omega-3 fatty acid not found in fish sources: alpha-linolenic acid, which is the basic building block for other omega-3s made in the body. Flaxseed oil, rich in alpha-linolenic acid, has provided greater protective effects against cardiovascular disease than linoleic acid-rich sunflower seed oil because of the ability of the linolenic acid to decrease the tendency of platelets to aggregate. Alpha linolenic acid is a precursor of EPA, shown to be beneficial in coronary heart disease, hypertension and inflammatory disorders. Linoleic acid is an antagonist of the process that converts alpha-linolenic acid to EPA.

## FORMULA FOR DISASTER

Omega-3 fatty acids are essential to proper vision and brain development in the newborn and are available to the fetus in the womb and to the newborn through breast milk. The brain, which develops rapidly in infants, is especially sensitive to deficiencies in essential fatty acids. For DHA, an omega-3 derivative, levels are crucial during the first months of life for development of visual acuity. Breast milk contains thirty times more DHA than formula.

The breast milk of nursing mothers, unfortunately, often contains high levels of trans fatty acids and low omega-3 content because of poor diets. Studies show that trans fatty acids in the diets of pregnant and nursing women reach the fetus and breast-fed baby and affect birth weight and subsequent growth. As reported in the British medical journal *The Lancet* (1995;345:1107-1108), essential fatty acid metabolism is adversely affected by trans fatty acids. Prepared infant formulas contain trans fatty acids. They also contain high omega-6 content compared to omega-3, and imbalance in fatty acids that can lead to future impairment of the infant's immune system.

Although breast milk has large quantities of fat, saturated fat and cholesterol, these fats are exactly what an infant needs for growth and development. These fats are also more digestible, producing less colic. The unique fat composition of breast milk (over 200 different fats), as well as the content of many other key nutrients, will tell you that cow's milk is for baby cows—human breast milk is for human babies.

Researchers supplemented formulas of preterm infants with marine oil as a source of DHA and compared results to other infants fed formulas without marine oil. They concluded that marine-oil-supplemented formula improved visual acuity of preterm infants through four months of age by improving DHA status.

## THE SEEDS OF GOOD HEALTH

Unsaturated oils derived from seeds are also excellent sources of essential fatty acids. Grape seed, once thought to be a mediocre oil, is now known to be an excellent source of proanthocyanadins, a special class of bioflavonoids with antioxidant properties (for information on these compounds, see Volume I of this series, *The Antioxidants*).

Hemp seed, the twin of flaxseed (see above) also contains high levels of alpha-linolenic acid, as well as linoleic acid and gamma-linolenic acid. No other common seed oil contains the gamma form of linolenic acid.

Black currant seed contains omega-3 and omega-6 fatty acids including gamma-linolenic acid. Borage seed, high in gamma-linolenic acid, has been used to treat arthritis, allergies, multiple sclerosis, cancer and PMS.

## BUTTER IS BETTER

We have learned that trans fatty acids disrupt the metabolism and function of the essential fatty acids, worsen essential fatty acid deficiencies, and contribute to heart disease. As early as 1956, medical journals such as *The Lancet* predicted that hydrogenation could turn out to be a contributor of heart disease. Their words fell on deaf ears.

It's estimated Americans consume 8 to 13 grams of trans fat daily. When researchers at Harvard University measured the trans-fat content of some restaurant and store-bought foods they found that four ounces of french fries contained 3.43 grams, one Danish pastry contained 3.03 grams, and one piece of cake or pie, about one gram of trans fat. Vegetable shortening and stick margarine contained about 0.6 grams per teaspoon, while the same amount of tub margarine contained 0.27 grams (*New England Journal of Medicine,* Dec. 23, 1993).

Among the recent studies implicating trans fats in coronary artery disease was one of nearly 90,000 women conducted by Dr. Walter

Willett and his colleagues at Harvard and published in 1993 in *The Lancet.* It found that those women who ate the most foods high in trans fats (especially margarine) had a more than 50 percent higher risk of heart disease than women who ate these fats rarely. Dr. Willett has estimated that the partially hydrogenated vegetable oils used to make margarine (as well as many cookies, crackers, and other processed foods) are responsible for more than 30,000 of the country's annual deaths from heart disease.

Nutrition labels are misleading, explains Dr. Willett, since they don't have to specify how much trans fat is in the foods. In fact, the chemical structure of some trans fatty acid forms allows them to be classified as "unsaturated" (although they are unnaturally unsaturated) leading consumers to believe that they are purchasing a healthy item. This omission may actually encourage food processors to increase their use of trans fats, according to Dr. Willett, since unlike the saturated fats they replace, the trans fats remain invisible on the new labels.

Trans fatty acids, again the culprit, were reported in the journal, *Circulation* (1994;89:94-101) to increase the risk of myocardial infarction by more than three times in people who consumed more than 2.5 pats of margarine per day. Butter, which does not contain trans fatty acids, did not significantly increase the risk. Previously, the Nurses' Health Study of 85,000 nurses found that margarine (as well as fried fast foods, cake, and cookies containing margarine and other trans fats) increased myocardial infarction risk, said Dr. Charles Hennekens, professor of medicine at Harvard.

## WASH IT DOWN WITH RED WINE

Results of a large European study (EURAMIC) also support the idea that trans fatty acids increase the risk of myocardial infarction. However, risks were different from one country to the next. In Norway, Finland and the U.S., high levels of trans fatty acids in fat tissue were associated with a higher risk of myocardial infarction than in Spain and Russia. Investigators found that the difference was in the amount of alcohol in the diet, higher in populations in Spain and Russia. The propensity of trans fatty acids to increase blood clots was offset by the ability of alcohol to decrease such clotting.

## CLOGGING THE PIPES

Edward N. Siguel M.D., Ph.D., and Robert H. Lerman M.D., Ph.D., of the Boston University Medical Center in Massachusetts, found that people with coronary artery disease have a much higher level of trans-fatty acids in their blood than those who do not show any evidence of heart disease. The study, published in the April 15, 1993 issue of *The American Journal of Cardiology,* confirms previous reports showing that trans-fatty acids increase low-density lipoprotein (LDL) cholesterol, the harmful kind, while decreasing high-density lipoprotein (HDL) cholesterol, the beneficial kind.

The researchers recommended that persons at risk for coronary artery disease with above-average plasma levels of trans-fatty acids should substantially modify their diets to eat less trans-fatty acids which have no known nutritional value.

An earlier study by Ronald P. Mensink, Ph.D., and Martijn B. Katan, in *The New England Journal of Medicine* in 1990, found that women who eat four or more teaspoons of margarine daily have a 50 percent greater risk of developing heart disease than women who eat margarine only once a month, with six or more teaspoons increasing the risk to 70 percent.

## MORE GOOD FAT EVIDENCE

More evidence is accumulating that some of the other oils and "fat partners" play key roles in promoting optimal health.

Lipoic acid, also called thioctic acid, has been used for the treatment of diabetic polyneuropathy in Europe. Researchers at the University College London Medical School found that lipoic acid can chelate copper ions that contribute to free-radical induced damage in blood cells.

Lipoic acid also works synergistically with vitamin C and with glutathione to protect blood cells from oxidative damage. The protective antioxidant effect is exerted directly outside the cells as free radicals are inactivated. Brewer's yeast is a good source of lipoic acid.

## THREE, SIX, NINE—OILS ARE JUST FINE

Finding the right balance of essential fatty acids is important. Researchers believe that a one-to-one ratio of omega-3s to the omega-6s (found primarily in vegetable oils like corn, safflower or sunflower) may be important in preventing heart disease.

Omega-3s and omega-6s continually compete for control of important biochemical reactions in the body. When omega-6s win the battle, it can lead to an overproduction of hormone-like substances called prostaglandins and leukotrienes. These compounds, in large amounts, can disrupt the immune system, initiate the build-up of plaque formations on artery walls, form blood clots and trigger dangerously irregular heart rhythms.

Currently, the ratio in the American diet is about ten to one (10 omega-6s to one omega-3), a level some experts say is a dangerous oversupply of omega-6 fatty acids. Researchers have found that eating fish two or three times a week improves the ratio of omega-3 to omega-6 fatty acids in the diet. You can also shift your ratio in the right direction by going easy on salad dressings, margarine, mayonnaise and vegetable oils other than olive and canola.

## DON'T FORGET THE MUFAs

Olive oil, although it contains only small amounts of the essential fatty acids linoleic and alpha-linolenic acid, has beneficial effects on health. It contains about 75 percent of the non-essential monounsaturated fatty acid (MUFA), oleic acid. Oleic acid is a member of the omega-9 family.

Oleic acid is also found in almond, peanut, pistachio, pecan, canola, avocado, hazelnut, cashew, and macadamia oils, as well as in plant and animal cells. This fatty acid helps keep our arteries flexible, reducing the risk of heart disease.

In addition to the benefits of monounsaturation discussed in the introduction to this book, there are also minor components in olive oil that enhance its health-giving properties. Olive oil contains beta-carotene, vitamin E, chlorophyll (rich in magnesium), and phytosterols that protect against cholesterol absorption from foods, and are all heart-healthy components.

Results from a study reported in the *Journal of the National Cancer Institute,* January 18, 1995, indicate that olive oil may prevent breast cancer. A look at the diets and the rate of breast cancer in 2,368 women in Greece suggests that women who used olive oil more than once a day had a 25-percent lower risk of breast cancer than women who used that fat less often. "I wouldn't suggest replacing fats with just any monounsaturated fats," says study co-author Dimitrios Trichopoulos, M.D., of the Harvard School of Public Health. "There may be something more in olive oil."

Olive oil also reduces the production of cholesterol-containing gallstones, contains triterpenic acids that have healing and anti-inflammatory effects, and contains phenolic compounds with antioxidant properties.

## FAT FACTS

- The normal brain is 60 percent fat. These fats are made from the omega-3 and omega-6 essential fatty acids which provide the fluidity needed for impulses to travel throughout the brain.
- When whole grain is milled to make white flour, the part discarded contains the germ, a good source of essential fatty acids, vitamin E and other vitamins and minerals.
- Hydrogenation of oils destroys the omega fatty acids. Omega-3 fatty acids are especially vulnerable to becoming rancid because they are unsaturated. A high degree of unsaturation is good for us but bad for shelf life. Guess who wins?

- Trans fatty acids are imposters—they fool cells into thinking they are useful for cell function, crowding out the real fatty acids. Trans fatty acids actually increase the need for essential fatty acids, while still providing calories.
- Trans fatty acids get stuck in muscles, liver, spleen, kidneys, adrenal glands and the heart, interfering with function of these structures.
- Many infants that died of sudden infant death syndrome (SIDS) were drinking formulas that lacked omega-3 fatty acids. Breast milk contains about 30 times more docosahexaenoic acid, an essential omega-3 fatty acid, than formula.
- Sixty-eight percent of people die from three conditions related to degenerative diseases that involve fats: cardiovascular disease (43.8 percent), cancer (22.4 percent) and diabetes (1.8 percent).
- Frying and deep-frying foods uses up natural antioxidants in oils such as vitamin E and carotenes that protect oils by preventing lipid peroxidation (rancidity). Frying also produces free radicals that further contribute to rancidity (antioxidants stop free radical reactions). Frying also produces trans fatty acids and scores of other unnatural breakdown products with unknown effects on health.

## THE FAT FUTURE

### A THIEF IN FAT'S CLOTHING

Did you expect the Food and Drug Administration or the major food manufacturers to start substituting the good fats and oils for those that are bad for us? They made a feeble attempt a decade ago when they started cooking french fries in vegetable oil instead of saturated beef tallow or tropical oils. McDonald's and other chains complied . . . well, almost. Many switched to vegetable shortening which is hydrogenated or partially hydrogenated. "Well, it's oil when it's in the fryer," said a Burger King spokesperson. So from beef tallow which contains about 4 percent trans fatty acids, the chains went to partially hydrogenated soybean oil with about 42 percent. Doughnuts previously fried in lard containing no trans fatty acids also got "transed."

What was next on the agenda of the corporate/government machine? Fake fat. Food manufacturers have always wanted to cash in on our obsession with fat. In 1990, the NutraSweet Company marketed Simplesse, a fat substitute. It is made from a whey protein concentrate, containing about one-tenth the calories of regular fat. So far it has been a disappointment. It cannot be used for frying at high temperatures. NutraSweet used it in their ice cream product, Simple Pleasures, until last year. Now, they only sell Simplesse to other food manufacturers.

Now things have gotten worse. In early 1996, the Food and Drug Administration approved Procter & Gamble's fat substitute, called olestra, for marketing. The company discovered it twenty-five years ago. A combination of table sugar, edible fats and oils that tastes, smells and cooks like natural fat, it is calorie-free. This is because its molecules are too large to be digested and simply pass through the intestines. Sounds too good to be true? Well, you are right. Besides causing intestinal upset such as diarrhea, olestra will absorb the fat-soluble vitamins from other foods in your diet. Thus, vitamins E, D, K and beta-carotene will take the fake fat rapid transit system right out of your body! The approval requires that companies who use the product fortify the foods with these vitamins and also carry a warning label that eating olestra may be harmful to your health. Cigarettes carry a similar warning, but that doesn't stop thousands of people from killing themselves.

## BUTTERING IT UP

A small Canadian company is working on a version of butter that tastes and cooks like the real thing but does not clog arteries. It has as much fat and calories as regular butter, but so far does not seem to raise cholesterol levels. Scientists at Harvard Medical School are currently testing it on volunteers in Boston. It could be ready for market in one to two years. According to the researchers, the fat molecules are "rearranged." No comprehensive safety study has yet been conducted but the company believes that the modified butter fat is harmless. As we have just seen with olestra, being harmful is not a prerequisite for disapproval by the Food and Drug Administration. *Caveat emptor*!

## DESIGNER GENES

Agronomists can now routinely introduce genes into many plant species. In the pipeline are new opportunities to genetically engineer plants to produce edible fats and oils with predefined fatty acid composition. A substantial amount of work is still required, however, before we see unsaturated coconut oil or monounsaturated corn oil.

## VITAMIN E EXTENDS ITS FAMILY

A class of compounds called tocotrienols, related to the tocopherols or vitamin E family, is now under investigation. While tocopherols are mostly found in soybean, corn and olive oils, it is the palm, rice bran and barley oils that are rich in tocotrienols.

Like their vitamin E cousins, tocotrienols have already been documented to be excellent antioxidants, having anti-cancer and cholesterol-reducing properties. They also travel with LDL cholesterol, protecting it from becoming oxidized and "bad."

## HAVE YOUR FAT AND EAT IT TOO

If this book has done what it was intended to do, you now have the knowledge that will ensure that you live a longer, happier and healthier life. You know that you can eat fats and oils, without incurring health hazards, providing you choose the good ones. When you look at a food label, the words "partially hydrogenated" will jump out at you with new meaning. You can protect your family, even your unborn fetus, from the ravages of trans fatty acids. You can enjoy your food more because it tastes good and is good for you. If you want to lose weight, you know that fat is an important dietary aid. Fats and oils are no longer your enemies, but are tools that can be used to engineer a healthier future for you and your loved ones. *The Good Fats and Oils* has empowered you to create a health plan you can live with for a long, long time.

## REFERENCES

Nielsen, G. L. *et al.* The Effects of Dietary Supplementation with n-3 Polyunsaturated Fatty Acids in Patients with Rheumatoid Arthritis: A Randomized, Double-Blind Trial. *European J. Clinical Investigation.* 1992;22 (10):687–691.

Ascherio, A., Rimm, E. B., Stampfer, M. J., Giovannucci, E, L., Willett, W. C. Dietary intake of marine omega-3 fatty acids, fish intake, and the risk of coronary disease among men. *The New England Journal of Medicine.* 1995;332:977.

Harris, W. S., Muzio, F. Fish oil reduces postprandial triglyceride concentrations without accelerating lipid-emulsion removal rates. *American Journal of Clinical Nutrition.* 1993;58:68.

Fish oils and angioplasty. *Executive Health*'s Good Health Report. April 1994;30:1.

Fish oil and colon cancer. (Diet and Cancer). *Nutrition Research Newsletter* Nov.-Dec. 1992;11:126.

Anti, M., *et al.* Effect of n-3 fatty acids on rectal mucosal cell proliferation in subjects at risk for colon cancer. *Gastroenterology.* 1992;103(3):883–391.

Fish oil for ulcerative colitis. *Prevention,* September, 1992;44:30.

Bairati, I., *et al.* Effects of a fish oil supplement on blood pressure and serum lipids in patients treated for coronary artery disease. *Canadian Journal of Cardiology.* 1992;8(1):41–46.

Giller, R. M., Matthews, K. *Natural Prescriptions.* New York: Carol Southern Books, 1994, pp. 15, 20, 199, 251, 290–294.

Nielsen, G. K., *et al.* The effects of dietary supplementation with N3 polyunsaturated fatty acids in patients with rheumatoid arthritis: A randomized, double-blind trial. *European Journal of Clinical Investigation.* 1992;22:687–691.

Seidelin, K.N., *et al.* N3 fatty acids in adipose tissue and coronary artery disease are inversely related. *American Journal of Clinical Nutrition.* 1992;55: 1117–1119.

Shahar, E., *et al.* Dietary N3 polyunsaturated fatty acids and smoking-related chronic obstructive pulmonary disease. *The New England Journal of Medicine.* 1994; 331(4):228–233.

Axelrod, L., Camuso, J., Williams, E., Kleinman, K., Briones, E., Schoenfeld, D. Effects of a small quantity of [omega]–3 fatty acids on cardiovascular risk factors in NIDDM. *Diabetes Care.* 1994;17(1):37–44.

Carlson, S.E., Werkman, S. H., Rhodes, P. G., Tolley, E. A. Visual-acuity development in healthy preterm infants: effect of marine-oil supplementation. *American Journal of Clinical Nutrition* 1993;58:35.

BeLieu, R. M. Evening Primrose Oil. *Obstet Gynecol Clin North Am.* 1994;21(3):461:477

Allman, M. A., Pena, M. M., Pang, D. *Eur. J. Clin. Nutr.* 1995;49(3):169–178.

Willett, W. C., Stampfer, M. J., Manson, J. E., *et al.* Intake of trans fatty acids and risk of coronary heart disease among women. *The Lancet* 1993;341:581-585.

Mensink, R. P., Katan, M. B. Effect of dietary trans fatty acids on high-density and low-density lipoprotein cholesterol levels in healthy subjects. *The New England Journal of Medicine.* 1990;327(7):439:445.

Siguel, E. N., Lerman, R. H. Trans-fatty acid patterns in patients with angiographically documented coronary artery disease. *The American Journal of Cardiology,* April 15, 1993.

Ou, P., Tritschler, H. J., Wolff, S. P. Thioctic (lipoic) acid: a therapeutical metal-chelating antioxidant? *Biochem. Pharmacol.* 1995;50(1):123-126.

Constantinescu, A., Tritschler, H., Packer, L. Alpha-lipoic acid protects against hemolysis of human erythrocytes induced by peroxyl radicals. *Biochem. Mol. Biol. Int.* 1994;33(4):669–679.

# The Culprit in Clogged Arteries Is Oxidation, Not Cholesterol

For a number of years now, research has been accumulating to suggest that many of the diseases that plague modern society, such as heart disease, arthritis and cancer, are primarily caused by oxidative destruction of the body's tissues. We need oxygen to burn our fuel and thus stay alive, but an excess amount of oxidation can cause severe damage to our cells.

We get old by oxidation. The wrinkling of aging skin is a result of protein cross-links, a product of oxidation. Cataracts in the eye are formed by rapid oxidation of the lens in the eye. The sturdy youthful tissues of the body, made largely of protein, are gradually torn apart by ongoing oxidative processes. And now there is new data to show that hardening of the arteries is also a product of oxidative damage, and not merely cholesterol.

## OXIDIZED CHOLESTEROL

A few years ago Dr. Thomas Carew of the University of California in San Diego tested the theory that oxidized cholesterol, and not ordinary cholesterol, was capable of inducing damage to artery walls. He studied a strain of rabbits that is highly prone to human type hardened arteries. One group of rabbits was given lovastatin, a medication now widely in use to lower cholesterol, and another group was given vitamin E, an antioxidant nutrient.

After seven months, there was a "striking decrease" in the number of cholesterol plaques in the blood vessels. The group receiving the vitamin E had less than half the amount of hardening that the other group showed. The finding is "an important new lead," said Dr. Michael Brown of the University of Texas Medical Center in Dallas. Dr. Brown and his associate won the Nobel prize in 1985 for their work on cholesterol.

As a result of these findings, dozens of new studies are now being started on human volunteers. There are no medications on the market that have been approved for antioxidant use. It will be 10 to 15 years before drug companies can develop compounds for FDA approval.

Instead of waiting for the pharmaceutical industry to come up with a new medication and risking side effects from these drugs, it is possible right now to achieve protection against oxidation by taking certain vitamins and minerals. Doctors in Canada, the Shute brothers, prescribed vitamin E for decades at their clinic for cardiovascular disease. Their patients responded with dramatically less heart trouble.

Another important antioxidant nutrient is vitamin C, which has such good antioxidant properties that it has even been used to preserve foods from spoilage. Vitamin B5 is another important antioxidant. Beta-carotene is not only an antioxidant, but also has very strong anti-cancer properties. Other nutrients with antioxidant activity include PABA, zinc, manganese, niacinamide, thiamin, selenium, germanium, vitamin A, gamma-linoleic acid and cystine.

## OXIDANTS TO AVOID

Avoiding oxidizing substances is another important way to protect against heart disease. Polyunsaturated fats and oils, commonly used in cooking, oxidize very rapidly and are then a risk for hardened arteries. These include corn oil, corn oil margarine, sunflower seed oil and safflower oil. Much less likely to oxidize are the oils rich in monounsaturates, such as olive oil, canola oil and peanut oil. Olive oil is much safer to cook with and has been shown to actually lower cholesterol.

Any oil that has been heated for an hour or more becomes highly oxidized and forms chemicals called lipid peroxides. These are highly reactive and dangerous substances, capable of causing not only heart disease but also cancer. Deep-fried foods of all kinds are thus a risk, since the cooking oil is typically used for hours, days or even weeks, by which time it is dangerously laden with peroxides. The safe alternative is pan-fried or stir-fried foods, which use fresh oil every time and cook the oil for only a few minutes.

## ENVIRONMENTAL FACTORS

Cigarette smoke is a very strong source of oxidizing chemicals. Also, exhaust fumes incite greatly increased production of oxidative metabolites, as do industrial waste gases. Many food additives also increase the danger, as do increased radiation from X-rays, high background radiation near nuclear plants, etc. Irradiated food contains many of these oxidized by-products. Strenuous exercise increases oxidative metabolism, and many athletes now take antioxidant nutritional supplements to enhance their performance and minimize the risk of injury from vigorous physical activity.

Under the proper supervision and with proper diet, the correct use of antioxidant nutrients can greatly reduce the risk of cardiac disease and other illnesses.*

THOMAS T. BRUNOSKI, M.D., M.S.

# Cholesterol's Role In Heart Disease Still Unclear; Tests Confusing, Contradictory

## *Drug-Free Means Of Reducing High Levels Include: Niacin, Vitamin C, Chromium, Rice Bran Oil, Magnesium And Calcium*

Even though the cholesterol controversy has been hotly debated for over 30 years, researchers are still in disagreement as to whether or not this fatlike substance is the real culprit in the development of cardiovascular disease. What is often overlooked in this simmering feud is that cholesterol is essential to life; that we use and replenish up to 2,000 mg of cholesterol daily; and the body, mostly in the liver, manufactures about two-thirds of our daily cholesterol intake, with the remaining one-third obtained from the diet.

To compound the problem, the researchers, with their extremely divergent opinions, have succeeded in confusing the general public and creating a vast library of misinformation. Part of the problem arises when the experts cannot agree on the distinction between total serum cholesterol, the amount of available high-density lipoprotein cholesterol (the so-called "good" kind) in relation to the amount of low-density lipoprotein cholesterol (considered the "bad" kind); the triglyceride reading; and numerous other factors, such as the amount of apolipoproteins, of which there are many kinds.

And researchers are not even in total agreement as to what constitutes a "normal" cholesterol level. Over the years that reading has continued to be

*For additional information on antioxidants, see *The Nutrition Superbook, Vol. I The Antioxidants* of this series.

dropped, and now a level of 200 mg/dl or below is considered ideal. There are potential problems if the count goes too low, and there is still confusion concerning the various ratios of HDL to LDL and so forth.

Numerous researchers have promoted a low-fat diet as one means of reducing cholesterol levels, and yet such a diet may predispose some patients to colon cancer, according to Moshe Shike, M.D., of New York's Memorial Sloan-Kettering Cancer Center, as reported in the June 13, 1990 issue of *Medical Tribune.*

An equally startling report was published in the September 6, 1990 issue of the same publication, which suggested that the lowering of serum cholesterol may be associated with a significant increase in deaths from suicide, accidents or violence.

The study showed an association between cholesterol reduction and higher mortality not related to illness, said Matthew F. Muldoon, M.D. of the University of Pittsburgh, one of the researchers.

Claude Lenfant, M.D., director of the National Heart, Lung and Blood Institute in Bethesda, Maryland, added that, "What has been observed for some time is that if you go to the lower extreme of serum cholesterol, you may find a reversal of the risk—the curve may go up again. But what we need to know is what is causing that reversal."

These suggestions do not seem too far-fetched when we realize that fat is necessary for the metabolizing of fat-soluble vitamins (A, D, E and K), for making sex hormones and the adrenal cortex, for maintaining body temperature, for providing a reserve source of energy, for repairing and replacing body cells, for forming a protective shield around nerves and muscles, for converting the sun's rays into vitamin D from cholesterol, and for furnishing about 30 percent of our daily calories, to name only a few.

## TEST OFTEN UNRELIABLE

The periodic testing of an individual's cholesterol level is recommended by many physicians, and yet the tests are often unreliable. For that reason, it is generally suggested that at least three tests be taken over a period of weeks or months and averaged. The test is so finicky that a reading taken in the morning can be entirely different from one that afternoon.

"There are still laboratories out there that do a very poor job of measuring cholesterol," according to Robert Olsen, M.D. of the State College of New York in Stony Brook in the April 4, 1990 issue of the *Medical Tribune.*

While many physicians continue to put their patients on low-fat diets, prescribe cholesterol-lowering drugs and drastically reduce dietary cholesterol intake, K. Fred Gey, M.D. and colleagues at the Institute of Biochemistry and Molecular Biology in Berne, Switzerland, rattled the scientific community by reporting that low blood levels of vitamin E are a more important risk factor than high cholesterol or high blood pressure for ischemic heart disease (IHD) mortality.

"Low levels of vitamin E in the blood are most predictive of IHD risk, even exceeding the predictive value of high cholesterol," stated *Medical Tribune* for February 7, 1990. "Cholesterol and high blood pressure had only a 'moderate' association with IHD mortality. Low vitamin E levels were found in 62 percent of men who died of IHD, and the combination of low vitamin E with high cholesterol, low vitamin A and high blood pressure raised the predictive value to 87 percent," Dr. Gey reported.

Since it is estimated that between 5 and 13 percent of the population has an inherited problem with cholesterol, cholesterol lowering procedures are, of course, in order for these patients. But the usual drugs prescribed have endless side effects, some of which can be life-threatening. For that reason, many physicians opt for dietary modifications and natural foods and supplements.

Vitamin B3 (niacin) is often effective in reducing cholesterol levels, unless the vitamin produces nausea, according to Jonathan V. Wright, M.D., in Dr. Wright's *Guide to Healing with Nutrition* (Keats, 1990). The so-called "niacin flush" can be uncomfortable for some people, but it passes and is not dangerous.

"Vitamin C can be very helpful, but it takes more than present in the usual multivitamin," Dr. Wright said. "Three grams (3,000 mg) daily—not all at once—is an 'average amount.' If you have a family or personal history of kidney stone, a lab test called '24-hour urine for oxalate' can help determine the maximum safe amount."

He added that lecithin, especially when combined with vitamin C, is useful in lowering total serum cholesterol. If you are using lecithin, Dr. Wright recommends a well-rounded tablespoon or six of the 19-grain capsules daily.

"Magnesium not only helps lower total serum cholesterol, but can raise HDL-cholesterol besides," he continued.

Between 600 and 1,000 mg of calcium daily can also lower total serum cholesterol, Dr. Wright said. He recommends a combination calcium and magnesium supplement.

## OTHER SUPPLEMENTS

"Chromium has been found to reduce atherosclerotic plaque (in experimental animals), lower total cholesterol and raise HDL-cholesterol (humans)," Dr. Wright added. "We've observed that 500 to 1,000 mcg daily of the picolinate or polynicotinate form usually does the job."

In several studies, pantethine, a metabolite of pantothenic acid, the B vitamin, has been shown to lower total serum cholesterol, he continued.

"L-carnitine lowers total cholesterol and raises HDL levels, too," Dr. Wright said. "While it's at it, it lowers triglycerides, another blood fat."

In a preliminary study using laboratory animals, Dr. Robert Nicolosi of the University of Lowell in Massachusetts told a symposium of the American Heart Association that rice bran oil lowered cholesterol levels by 30 percent without reducing HDL, according to *The New York Times,* January 15, 1991.

In volume 53 of the *American Journal of Clinical Nutrition,* 1991, researchers at the Upjohn Research Clinics in Kalamazoo, Michigan, report that beta-carotene, the precursor for vitamin A, raises beneficial HDL.

With all of the natural ways of reducing cholesterol and the other fats, it is still a mystery why so many physicians continue to use only drugs. As this brief review suggests, the possibilities of lowering dietary fats through natural means are virtually endless.

### BODY FAT AND CHOLESTEROL

People with big hips and trim waists have higher levels of high-density lipoprotein (HDL) cholesterol, the beneficial kind, than do those with potbellies, according to recent research. Fat around the hips tends to be subcutaneous fat, while fat around the waist is intraabdominal fat, which drains directly to the liver and may interfere with the organ's production of HDL, the researchers added. (*U.S. Pharmacist,* March 1990.)

# Essential Fats Help Relieve Diabetes and Osteoporosis

Exciting new research into the natural treatment and prevention of both diabetes and osteoporosis again brings to our attention the important role the essential fatty acids (EFAs) play in nearly every aspect of human health. The word "essential" means that we must get these dietary oils either in foods such as fish, grains, seeds or cold-pressed vegetable oils or from supplements such as fish oils, evening primrose oil, flaxseed oil, borage seed oil or black currant seed oil. Our body is not capable of making EFAs either at all or in sufficient quantities for good health.

The EFAs are linoleic acid (omega-6) and alpha-linolenic acid (omega-3). Omega-6 and omega-3 cannot be interconverted, that is, omega-6 cannot be made into omega-3 and omega-3 cannot be made into omega-6; therefore we need both omega-3 and omega-6 EFAs in our diet.

Historically, we have known about essential fatty acids for over 100 years. It is only in the last 20 years, however, that we have come to understand that dietary EFAs are important for a compelling new reason: they are building blocks for an important category of hormones called *prostanoids*. Prior to that time, we viewed essential fatty acids as necessary components of cell membranes and as a source of fuel (or calories).

Hormones are "control" molecules. They are produced in one location, travel in the body and have an effect in a second location. Endocrine hormones such as thyroxin (produced in the thyroid) and cortisone (produced in the adrenals) travel in our blood and have effects on tissues and organs in other parts of our body. Prostaglandin hormones, on the other hand, are "short distance" messenger molecules. They typically travel from one cell to the next cell and are most useful as a means for one cell in our body to communicate with another.

## DIABETES

The major essential fatty acid is linoleic acid (LA) also known as omega-6. The body needs to convert LA to gamma-linolenic acid (GLA). This conversion is facilitated by an enzyme called delta-6-desaturase. In diabetes, this enzyme is impaired and conversion of LA to GLA is compromised.

Many studies on diabetic animals have shown that they require higher amounts of linoleic acid than normal animals. This increased requirement for linoleic acid (LA ) results from the decreased conversion of LA to GLA. Since GLA and metabolites of GLA (such as dihomogammalinolenic acid—also called DGLA) are required for many metabolic reactions, excess LA (its precursor) is required to make enough GLA when the conversion is "sluggish." This metabolic block may be overcome by taking GLA directly as a dietary supplement and not depending on the conversion of LA to GLA. GLA supplements include evening primrose oil, black currant seed oil and borage seed oil.

When the various fatty acids were measured in the membranes of diabetics as opposed to non-diabetics, it was found that the amount of the GLA metabolic product DGLA in diabetics was one-half that of non-diabetics, whereas the linoleic acid concentration was the same or slightly higher. Thus the conclusion that conversion of linoleic acid to DGLA (a metabolic product of GLA) is compromised is further supported.

In a recent study in England, 111 patients with diabetic neuropathy were divided into two groups. One group received 12 capsules of evening primrose oil per day and the control group received no supplementation at all. The evening primrose oil was a source of gamma-linolenic acid (GLA). The results were consistent with previous studies on animals. In this study of people with diabetic neuropathy, there was consistent improvement in neurological systems in those who took the evening primrose oil capsules as compared to the control group which did not.

## OSTEOPOROSIS

Osteoporosis affects both men and women. Although we normally think of osteoporosis as a women's disease, one in four hip fractures occur in men. The following thus applies to both men and women.

Dietary calcium has one of two fates. Either it is absorbed into the bloodstream for potential utilization by bone, or it is excreted in feces. Fecal

SOURCES OF OMEGA-6 ESSENTIAL FATTY ACIDS

Evening primrose oil
Black currant seed oil
Borage seed oil
Most vegetable, seed or nut oils
Meat and dairy fats

SOURCES OF OMEGA-3 ESSENTIAL FATTY ACIDS

Flax seed oil
Fish oil
Leafy greens (small amounts)

excretion of dietary calcium runs a wide range from 20 to 80 percent of ingested calcium. Obviously, the more calcium that moves out of the GI tract into the bloodstream, the more beneficial the effect. When calcium is absorbed into the blood it again has one of two fates. Either it is deposited in bone, or it is excreted by kidneys and urination. Here, both omega-6 and omega-3 fatty acids help prevent osteoporosis each in a different way.

Omega-6 fatty acids (GLA) seem to improve calcium absorption from the gastrointestinal tract. This is the first important step in ensuring strong bones. Calcium needs to be absorbed from dietary calcium in the GI tract into the bloodstream for it to be accessible in building strong bones.

On the other hand, arachidonic acid (AA), an essential fatty acid derived only from meat and dairy fats, speeds up urinary calcium excretion. Omega-3 EFAs, mainly from fish oils, are antagonistic to arachidonic acid and metabolites made from arachidonic acid. It is therefore no surprise that the omega-3 EFAs prevent calcium excretion, thus insuring strong bones.

In this age of fat-obsession, the take-home message is loud and clear. It is not just the *quantity* but the *quality* of the fats we eat that impact on our health. A small amount of healthy fat derived from high quality vegetable, seed or nut oils plus regular consumption of fish and leafy green vegetables is essential to good health. On the other hand, for those at risk for or suffering from such health problems as diabetes or osteoporosis, supplementation with these essential fats is definitely worth considering.

NEIL S. ORENSTEIN, PH.D.

# Don't Flee the Friendly Fats—They're Needed for Full Health

## *Low-Fat Diets "Can Kill You," Hinder Growth, Promote Allergies; It's the Saturated Fats You Have to Shun*

Drawing on years of research and study. Dr. Erasmus claims that "the lack of essential fatty acids is the biggest single nutrient deficiency of our time." However, while Americans are starving their bodies of the health-giving oils found in fresh nuts, seeds (particularly flax and hemp), soybeans and fish, they are overdosing on the hard, saturated fats in meats and dairy products and the chemically altered fats in margarine and commercially hydrogenated oils. Erasmus sees this as a deadly combination.

Switching to a nutritionally correct, low-fat diet will not solve this problem, according to Erasmus. In fact, he says that "low-fat diets can kill you. They can stunt growth in children, promote food allergies and lower immune function." Erasmus points out that the proponents of low-fat diets often live in California, Florida, or other warm climates where less oil is needed. In cold climates, more oil is required for good health; Erasmus suggests that 15 to 20% of calories should come from fat in a health-supportive diet.

### HEALTHY FATS AND THEIR USES

But not just any fat will do. Following are Erasmus's guidelines for healthy fats and their uses:

✓ The fats must be rich in essential fatty acids (EFAs).

✓ They must have the proper balance of omega-3 and omega-6 fatty acids.

✓ They must be cold-pressed and protected from light, heat and oxidation.

✓ They must be fresh. EFA-rich oils deteriorate with time unless frozen solid.

✓ They must be packaged in amber glass bottles to protect them from light; oils and plastic are a bad combination.

✓ They must not be used for frying or high-temperature cooking and they must be kept refrigerated.

### FLAX OIL AGAINST BREAST CANCER

A study published in the *British Journal of Cancer* (70:1994) suggests that supplementing the diet with flaxseed oil, a substance rich in alpha-linolenic acid, may help prevent breast cancer, tumor invasiveness and/or metastasis. The adipose breast tissue of 121 women with initially localized breast cancer was examined at the time of surgery; those with positive axillary lymph node status and vascular invasion were found to have a low level of alpha-linolenic acid. After 31 months of follow-up, 21 patients, all with low levels of alpha-linolenic acid, developed metastases. Previous animal studies have shown that diets rich in linoleic or omega-6 fatty acids (corn oil, safflower oil) stimulate mammary tumor growth, while those rich in linolenic or omega-3 fatty acids (flaxseed oil) inhibit it. Flaxseed oil is also high in lignans which offer additional anticancer benefits.

Erasmus's oils of choice are hemp oil and flaxseed oil; these oils contain the "healthy fats" in the proper proportions which are vital for good health. He recommends one to three tablespoons a day to yield an optimum EFA intake for healthy people. Those suffering from degenerative conditions such as heart disease, cancer or arthritis may need more.

These oils may be taken by the spoonful or are easily incorporated into the diet. They can be used in salad dressings, added to protein shakes or mixed with yogurt, hot cereals, baked potatoes or steamed vegetables. When fresh, these oils have a lovely nutty flavor. Flax or hemp oil can be mixed in with equal parts of olive oil for Mediterranean dishes or with equal parts of sweet organic butter for a spread or vegetable topping. They should never be used as cooking oils, because light, oxygen and high temperatures break them down and make them toxic. Adding them to hot cooked food before serving is fine.

Fresh, whole, unroasted seeds and nuts are another source of the healing fats. They make a wonderful snack with a piece of fruit or can be sprinkled liberally over grains, legumes and vegetables.

## CUTTING BACK ON KILLER FATS

At the same time that one is adding the healing fats to the diet, it makes sense to cut back on what Erasmus dubs the "killer fats." They include:

- ✗ Hydrogenated or partially hydrogenated margarines, shortenings, vegetable oils or any products that contain them. These processed oils double the risk of heart attacks and interfere with liver function, insulin function and EFA function, to name just a few of their deleterious effects.
- ✗ Fried or deep-fried foods which can cause cancer and hardening of the arteries.
- ✗ Refined, deodorized, colorless, odorless, tasteless mass-market oils which can cause mutations.
- ✗ An excess of hard fats like butter, beef, pork, lamb and tropical fats which make platelets sticky, interfere with insulin receptors and EFA functions. A "little bit" of butter is okay for healthy people, according to Erasmus, but it should be avoided entirely by those with cancer, diabetes, or heart and artery disease.

So stock up on flaxseed oil, avoid processed foods that contain hydrogenated fats by becoming a careful reader, consume foods as close to their natural state as possible and remember that not all fats are equal as far as good health is concerned.

# APPENDICES

# APPENDIX A

## Amount of Fats in Some Popular Foods

(Percentages do not equal 100 percent.)

| Food | Total Fat | Unsaturated | Saturated |
|---|---|---|---|
| *Salad and Cooking Oils* | | | |
| Safflower | 100 | 87 | 10 |
| Sunflower | 100 | 84 | 11 |
| Corn | 100 | 81 | 13 |
| Cottonseed | 100 | 71 | 23 |
| Soybean | 100 | 75 | 14 |
| Sesame | 100 | 80 | 14 |
| Peanut | 100 | 76 | 18 |
| Olive | 100 | 83 | 11 |
| Coconut | 100 | 6 | 80 |
| *Vegetable Fats—shortening* | 100 | 46 | 23 |
| *Margarines—First ingredient on label* | | | |
| Safflower, tub | 80 | 66 | 11 |
| Corn oil, tub | 80 | 64 | 14 |
| Soybean oil, tub | 80 | 64 | 15 |
| Corn oil, stick | 80 | 62 | 15 |
| Soybean oil, stick | 80 | 65 | 15 |
| Cottonseed, partially hydrogenated | 80 | 65 | 16 |
| Butter | 81 | 29 | 46 |
| *Animal Fats* | | | |
| Poultry | 100 | 60 | 30 |
| Beef, lamb, pork | 100 | 50 | 46 |
| *Fish, Raw* | | | |
| Salmon | 9 | 6 | 2 |
| Mackerel | 13 | 7 | 5 |
| Herring, Pacific | 13 | 5 | 4 |
| Tuna | 5 | 3 | 2 |
| *Nuts* | | | |
| Walnuts, English | 64 | 50 | 4 |
| Walnuts, Black | 60 | 49 | 4 |
| Brazil | 67 | 49 | 13 |

| Food | Total Fat | Unsaturated | Saturated |
|---|---|---|---|
| Peanuts or peanut butter | 51 | 39 | 9 |
| Pecan | 65 | 72 | 6 |
| *Egg yolk* | 31 | 15 | 10 |
| *Avocado* | 16 | 9 | 3 |

Arthur L. Frank, *Bestways,* November 1975.

# APPENDIX B

## Comparison of Dietary Fats

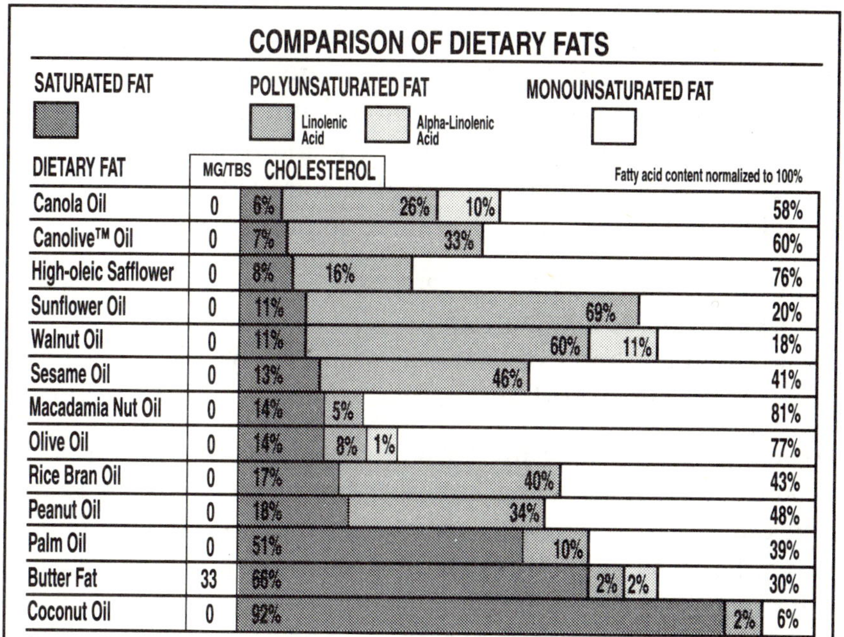


Courtesy of Loriva Supreme Foods, Hauppauge, NY

## APPENDIX C

# Structure and Function of Lipoic Acid

The chemical structure of lipoic acid gives it unique capabilities. It consists of a relatively small, eight-member chain having two sulfur atoms, one attached to the sixth carbon atom and the other sulfur atom attached to the eighth carbon atom, with the sulfurs also linked to each other which results in a ring. The molecular weight of lipoic acid is 206. The high-energy sulfur atoms are largely responsible for lipoic acid's ability to function in three important ways:

1. As a coenzyme in the energy process,
2. As a powerful antioxidant, and
3. As a chelator to remove excess iron and copper, and toxic metals such as cadmium, lead and mercury.

We know how unique the structure of the compound is, but we don't know very much about how this complex compound is assembled in the body, so we don't know what the limiting factors are for its biosynthesis. When I asked Dr. Jim Clark of the Henkel Corporation, he suggested that it is synthesized from an eight-carbon carboxylic acid called octanoic acid. Dr. Clark also suggested that the sulfur atoms come from cysteine, a sulfur-containing amino acid, but the exact chemical mechanism and the factors that control the synthesis are not known yet. This suggests to me that a dietary deficiency of sulfur-containing amino acids would limit the production of lipoic acid, but there are other nutritional factors and diseases that also interfere with lipoic acid production.

As I mentioned in the chapter on lipoic acid, the body does not make enough lipoic acid for optimal health. The optimal level of lipoic acid varies from person to person depending on biochemical individuality, lifestyle, and especially how much exercise and oxidative stress they experience. Age, disease and environmental conditions that increase oxidative stress can cause a deficiency in lipoic acid, so that the body can't make enough to meet all its metabolic and antioxidant needs. There is a lot of evidence that the body makes barely enough for its metabolic needs and does not produce enough for optimal antioxidant needs. The additional lipoic acid needed for antioxidant functions must come from dietary sources, including supplements. In some stressful situations it is necessary to get lipoic acid for both optimal metabolic function and antioxidant functions via the diet. This, again, is why lipoic acid is considered "conditionally essential."

## BOTH WATER- AND FAT-SOLUBLE

One of the reasons that lipoic acid is so versatile is that it can go virtually anywhere in the body to function. It is a rare nutrient in that it is compatible with—and soluble in—both water-based and fat-based components of the body. There are only two systems of solubility—polar and nonpolar. This translates into plain English as water-soluble and fat-soluble.

Lipoic acid's dual solubility is a main reason that it is sometimes referred to as a universal antioxidant, as well as the metabolic antioxidant. It is not as water-soluble as vitamin C, but it is much more water-soluble than vitamin E. Its degree of water-solubility and fat-solubility allows lipoic acid entry into all body systems. The main reason for this dual solubility is the size of the molecule. With a molecular weight of 206, it is larger than ascorbic acid (molecular weight of 176) but much smaller than vitamin E (molecular weight of 431).

A second factor is the functionality of the molecule. It does contain a carboxylic acid end-group, and that has a tendency to make it more soluble in water than vitamin E. At the same time it has more carbon atoms than vitamin C and that makes it more soluble in lipid compartments.

## THE SULFUR ATOMS ARE THE KEY

The chemical structure of lipoic acid is a simple molecule having a "backbone" of eight carbon atoms. Nature, instead of adding a hydroxyl group to form a monophenol nutrient like vitamin E, or adding several hydroxyl groups similar to bioflavonoids, adds two sulfur atoms and links them together. Sulfur atoms have a lot to do with lipoic acid's function as a coenzyme.

Lipoic acid is a cofactor in what is called a multienzyme complex. The lipoic acid itself is bound to a very complex enzyme which is a high-molecular weight protein. As such, it is not consumed when it is serving as a metabolic cofactor but is continually regenerated.

The process gets rather complex. But when lipoic acid is in its role of a metabolic coenzyme, the carboxylic acid end-group anchors it to the enzyme through formation of a chemical bond called an "amide linkage" or a "peptide linkage."

The sulfur atoms are critical to the action of lipoic acid as an enzyme, and also keys to lipoic acid being a powerful and versatile antioxidant.

## SULFUR MAKES LIPOIC ACID A POWERFUL ANTIOXIDANT

Adding to the versatility conveyed by lipoic acid's dual solubility is the fact that it also cycles between its oxidized and reduced forms, which are both powerful biological antioxidants. The fact that lipoic acid has a ring structure having a sulfur-sulfur linkage that can split, breaking the ring, and allow hydrogen to be added to the sulfur atoms has much to do with the antioxidant function of the molecule. The oxidation potential between the sulfur-sulfur bond and the sulfur-hydrogen bond is such as to allow easy interconversion under physiological conditions. The tissues can quite easily convert lipoic acid, which has a sulfur-sulfur bond, to dihydrolipoic acid, which has cleaved that sulfur-sulfur bond and replaced it with two sulfur-hydrogen bonds.

In allowing this hydrogen addition to the sulfur atoms, lipoic acid can cycle back and forth between the two forms—lipoic acid and dihydrolipoic acid. This is called "redox cycling." Redox cycling is simply the interconversion of an oxidized form of the material to a reduced form and back again. In some materials, the oxidation or reduction is irreversible. But the reduction and oxidation of lipoic acid is quite reversible; it can sit there and switch from one to the other. This is a real advantage because it allows it to act as a carrier, as a transfer agent for electrons from one compound to another.

The two forms have different chemical functionalities and can react in different ways with other materials. Compounds that supply hydrogen atoms or electrons in chemical reactions are called reducing agents. Oxidizing agents are compounds that receive hydrogen atoms or electrons. The primary difference is the fact that the reduced form—the dihydrolipoic acid—is a much stronger reducing agent and it is capable of regenerating vitamin C and vitamin E from their oxidized forms.

## SULFUR HELPS REMOVE TOXIC METALS

It is apparent that lipoic acid is itself a versatile and direct antioxidant. However, there is still more to its antioxidant protective actions. It also has an indirect action via its ability to remove toxic metals and excessive minerals.

## SUMMARY

1. Lipoic acid has a unique structure that gives it many special actions.
2. Lipoic acid is both water-soluble and fat-soluble.
3. Its sulfur atoms are the key to its coenzyme function, antioxidant function and chelating function.
4. Lipoic acid is not technically a vitamin, but it is so important to the

body that the body makes some. However, lipoic acid is "conditionally essential," meaning that most people may not make enough in their bodies for optimal health.

5. Lipoic acid is well-absorbed and transported into the cells where it does its many jobs.

RICHARD PASSWATER, PH.D.

# APPENDIX D

# Table on the Fatty Acid and Cholesterol Content of Selected Foods

| Food item | Common Measure | Weight | Food energy | Energy from fat | Total fat | Fatty acids: Saturated | Fatty acids: Monounsaturated | Fatty acids: Polyunsaturated | Cholesterol |
|---|---|---|---|---|---|---|---|---|---|
| | | g | kcal | kcal | g | g | g | g | mg |
| **Dairy and Egg Products** | | | | | | | | | |
| Cheese: | | | | | | | | | |
| American | 1 oz | 28 | 106 | 78 | 8.9 | 5.6 | 2.5 | 0.3 | 27 |
| Blue | 1 oz | 28 | 100 | 72 | 8.2 | 5.3 | 2.2 | 0.2 | 21 |
| Camembert | 1 oz | 28 | 85 | 61 | 6.9 | 4.3 | 2.0 | 0.2 | 20 |
| Cheddar | 1 oz | 28 | 114 | 83 | 9.4 | 6.0 | 2.7 | 0.3 | 30 |
| Cottage: | | | | | | | | | |
| Creamed, 4 percent fat: | | | | | | | | | |
| Large curd | 1 cup | 225 | 232 | 89 | 10.1 | 6.4 | 2.9 | 0.3 | 34 |
| Small curd | 1 cup | 210 | 217 | 84 | 9.5 | 6.0 | 2.7 | 0.3 | 31 |
| Lowfat, 1 percent fat | 1 cup | 226 | 164 | 20 | 2.3 | 1.5 | 0.7 | 0.1 | 10 |
| Uncreamed, dry curd, less than 1/2 percent fat | 1 cup | 145 | 123 | 5 | 0.6 | 0.4 | 0.2 | Tr[1] | 10 |
| Cream | 1 oz | 28 | 99 | 87 | 9.9 | 6.2 | 2.8 | 0.4 | 31 |
| Mozzarella, made with part skim milk | 1 oz | 28 | 72 | 40 | 4.5 | 2.9 | 1.3 | 0.1 | 16 |
| Muenster | 1 oz | 28 | 104 | 75 | 8.5 | 5.4 | 2.5 | 0.2 | 27 |
| Parmesan, grated | 1 tbsp | 5 | 23 | 13 | 1.5 | 1.0 | 0.4 | Tr | 4 |
| Ricotta, made with part skim milk | 1 oz | 28 | 39 | 19 | 2.2 | 1.4 | 0.7 | 0.1 | 9 |
| Swiss | 1 oz | 28 | 107 | 69 | 7.8 | 5.0 | 2.1 | 0.3 | 26 |
| Cream: | | | | | | | | | |
| Half-and-half (cream and milk) | 1 tbsp | 15 | 20 | 15 | 1.7 | 1.1 | 0.5 | 0.1 | 6 |
| Heavy, whipping, unwhipped | 1 tbsp | 15 | 52 | 49 | 5.6 | 3.5 | 1.6 | 0.2 | 21 |
| Light, coffee, or table | 1 tbsp | 15 | 29 | 25 | 2.9 | 1.8 | 0.8 | 0.1 | 10 |
| Cream, sour, cultured | 1 tbsp | 12 | 26 | 22 | 2.5 | 1.6 | 0.7 | 0.1 | 5 |
| Cream products, imitaiton (made with vegetable fat): | | | | | | | | | |
| Coffee whitener | | | | | | | | | |
| Liquid, frozen (contains coconut or palm kernel oil) | 1/2 fl oz | 15 | 20 | 13 | 1.5 | 1.4 | Tr | Tr | 0 |
| Powdered (contains coconut or palm kernel oil) | 1 tbsp | 6 | 6 | 33 | 19 | 2.1 | 1.8 | Tr | Tr |

| Food item | Common Measure | Weight | Food energy | Energy from fat | Total fat | Fatty acids: Saturated | Fatty acids: Monounsaturated | Fatty acids: Polyunsaturated | Cholesterol |
|---|---|---|---|---|---|---|---|---|---|
| | | g | kcal | kcal | g | g | g | g | mg |
| Dessert toppings (nondairy): | | | | | | | | | |
| Powdered, made with whole milk | 1 tbsp | 4 | 8 | 4 | 0.5 | 0.4 | Tr | Tr | Tr |
| Pressurized | 1 tbsp | 4 | 11 | 8 | 0.9 | 0.8 | 0.1 | Tr | 0 |
| Milk, fluid: | | | | | | | | | |
| Buttermilk, cultured | 1 cup | 245 | 99 | 19 | 2.2 | 1.3 | 0.6 | 0.1 | 9 |
| Whole (3.3 percent fat) | 1 cup | 244 | 150 | 72 | 8.2 | 5.1 | 2.4 | 0.3 | 33 |
| Lowfat (2 percent fat) | 1 cup | 245 | 125 | 41 | 4.7 | 2.9 | 1.4 | 0.2 | 18 |
| Lowfat (1 percent fat) | 1 cup | 245 | 104 | 21 | 2.4 | 1.5 | 0.7 | 0.1 | 10 |
| Nonfat, skim | 1 cup | 245 | 90 | 5 | 0.6 | 0.4 | 0.2 | Tr | 5 |
| Milk beverages: | | | | | | | | | |
| Eggnog | 1 cup | 254 | 342 | 167 | 19.0 | 11.3 | 5.7 | 0.9 | 118 |
| Shakes, thick, vanilla | 1 container | 313 | 350 | 84 | 9.5 | 5.9 | 2.7 | 0.4 | 37 |
| Milk desserts, frozen: | | | | | | | | | |
| Ice cream: | | | | | | | | | |
| Regular (about 10 percent fat) | 1 cup | 133 | 269 | 126 | 14.3 | 8.9 | 4.1 | 0.5 | 59 |
| Rich (about 16 percent fat) | 1 cup | 148 | 349 | 208 | 23.7 | 14.7 | 6.8 | 0.9 | 88 |
| Ice milk: | | | | | | | | | |
| Hardened (about 4.3 percent fat) | 1 cup | 131 | 184 | 49 | 5.6 | 3.5 | 1.6 | 0.2 | 18 |
| Soft serve (about 2.6 percent fat) | 1 cup | 175 | 223 | 40 | 4.6 | 2.9 | 1.3 | 0.2 | 13 |
| Sherbet (about 2 percent fat) | 1 cup | 193 | 270 | 33 | 3.8 | 2.4 | 1.1 | 0.1 | 14 |
| Yogurt: | | | | | | | | | |
| With added milk solids: | | | | | | | | | |
| Made with lowfat milk | 1 container | 227 | 194 | 25 | 2.8 | 1.8 | 0.8 | 0.1 | 11 |
| Made with nonfat milk | 1 container | 227 | 127 | 4 | 0.4 | 0.3 | 0.1 | Tr | 4 |
| Without added milk solids, made with whole milk | 1 container | 227 | 139 | 65 | 7.4 | 4.8 | 2.0 | 0.2 | 29 |
| Eggs, large: | | | | | | | | | |
| Hard-cooked, shell removed | 1 egg | 50 | 79 | 51 | 5.6 | 1.7 | 2.2 | 0.7 | 218 |
| Fried in butter | 1 egg | 46 | 94 | 66 | 7.2 | 2.7 | 2.7 | 0.8 | 223 |
| Scrambled (milk added) in butter; or omelet | 1 egg | 64 | 107 | 72 | 8.0 | 3.2 | 2.9 | 0.8 | 226 |
| **Fats, Oils, and Related Products** | | | | | | | | | |
| Fats(solid at room temperature): | | | | | | | | | |
| Butter | 1 tbsp | 14 | 102 | 102 | 11.4 | 7.1 | 3.3 | 0.4 | 31 |
| Lard | 1 tbsp | 13 | 116 | 116 | 12.8 | 5.0 | 5.8 | 1.4 | 12 |
| Margarine, diet (about 40 percent fat), tub[2] | 1 tbsp | 14 | 50 | 50 | 5.7 | 1.2 | 2.4 | 2.1 | 0 |
| Margarine, regular (at least 80 percent fat): | | | | | | | | | |
| Stick: | | | | | | | | | |
| Corn oil | 1 tbsp | 14 | 102 | 102 | 11.4 | 2.0 | 5.5 | 3.4 | 0 |
| Soybean oil | 1 tbsp | 14 | 102 | 102 | 11.4 | 2.4 | 5.4 | 3.0 | 0 |
| Tub: | | | | | | | | | |
| Corn oil | 1 tbsp | 14 | 102 | 102 | 11.4 | 2.0 | 4.5 | 4.4 | 0 |
| Soybean oil | 1 tbsp | 14 | 102 | 102 | 11.4 | 1.8 | 5.1 | 3.9 | 0 |

| Food item | Common Measure | Weight | Food energy | Energy from fat | Total fat | Fatty acids: Saturated | Fatty acids: Monounsaturated | Fatty acids: Polyunsaturated | Cholesterol |
|---|---|---|---|---|---|---|---|---|---|
| | | g | kcal | kcal | g | g | g | g | mg |
| Margarine, spread (about 60 percent fat): | | | | | | | | | |
| Stick[2] | 1 tbsp | 14 | 78 | 78 | 8.7 | 2.1 | 3.6 | 2.7 | 0 |
| Tub[2] | 1 tbsp | 14 | 78 | 78 | 8.7 | 1.8 | 4.5 | 2.1 | 0 |
| Shortening (animal and vegetable fat) | 1 tbsp | 13 | 115 | 115 | 12.8 | 5.2 | 5.7 | 1.4 | 7 |
| Shortening (vegetable fat) | 1 tbsp | 13 | 113 | 113 | 12.8 | 3.2 | 5.7 | 3.3 | 0 |
| Tallow, edible | 1 tbsp | 13 | 116 | 116 | 12.8 | 6.4 | 5.3 | 0.5 | 14 |
| Oils (liquid at room temperature): | | | | | | | | | |
| Coconut | 1 tbsp | 14 | 117 | 117 | 13.6 | 11.8 | 0.8 | 0.2 | 0 |
| Corn | 1 tbsp | 14 | 120 | 120 | 13.6 | 1.7 | 3.3 | 8.0 | 0 |
| Olive | 1 tbsp | 14 | 119 | 119 | 13.5 | 1.8 | 9.9 | 1.1 | 0 |
| Palm | 1 tbsp | 14 | 120 | 120 | 13.6 | 6.7 | 5.0 | 1.3 | 0 |
| Palm kernel | 1 tbsp | 14 | 117 | 117 | 13.6 | 11.1 | 1.5 | 0.2 | 0 |
| Peanut | 1 tbsp | 14 | 119 | 119 | 13.5 | 2.3 | 6.2 | 4.3 | 0 |
| Rapeseed (canola) | 1 tbsp | 14 | 120 | 120 | 13.6 | 0.9 | 7.6 | 4.5 | 0 |
| Safflower | 1 tbsp | 14 | 120 | 120 | 13.6 | 1.2 | 1.6 | 10.1 | 0 |
| Soybean oil | 1 tbsp | 14 | 120 | 120 | 13.6 | 2.0 | 3.2 | 7.9 | 0 |
| Sunflower | 1 tbsp | 14 | 120 | 120 | 13.6 | 1.4 | 2.7 | 8.9 | 0 |
| Related products: | | | | | | | | | |
| Mayonnaise | 1 tbsp | 14 | 99 | 99 | 11.0 | 1.6 | 3.1 | 5.7 | 6 |
| Peanut butter | 1 tbsp | 16 | 95 | 73 | 8.3 | 1.7 | 3.8 | 2.4 | 0 |
| **Fish, Shellfish, Meat, Poultry, and Related Products** | | | | | | | | | |
| Fish: | | | | | | | | | |
| Canned: | | | | | | | | | |
| Salmon, sockeye, water pack, drained solids | 3 oz | 85 | 130 | 46 | 6.2 | 1.4 | 1.2 | 1.9 | 37 |
| Sardines, Pacific, in tomato sauce, drained solids | 3 oz | 85 | 151 | 92 | 10.2 | 2.6 | 3.1 | 3.7 | 52 |
| Tuna, light, oil pack, drained solids | 3 oz | 85 | 169 | 63 | 7.0 | 1.3 | 2.5 | 2.5 | 15 |
| Cooked, dry heat: | | | | | | | | | |
| Flounder or sole (a lean fish) | 3 oz | 85 | 99 | 12 | 1.3 | 0.3 | 0.3 | 0.4 | 58 |
| Salmon, (fatty fish) | 3 oz | 85 | 183 | 84 | 9.3 | 1.6 | 4.5 | 2.0 | 74 |
| Shellfish: | | | | | | | | | |
| Canned: | | | | | | | | | |
| Crabmeat, steamed, pasturized | 3 oz | 85 | 84 | 9 | 1.0 | 0.2 | 0.2 | 0.4 | 76 |
| Shrimp, canned, dry pack | 3 oz | 85 | 102 | 8 | 0.9 | 0.3 | 0.2 | 0.6 | 147 |
| Raw: | | | | | | | | | |
| Clams, unspecified | 3 oz | 85 | 63 | 7 | 0.8 | 0.1 | 0.1 | 0.2 | 29 |
| Oyseters, Eastern (6 medium) | 3 oz | 85 | 59 | 19 | 2.1 | 0.5 | 0.2 | 0.6 | 47 |
| Meat: | | | | | | | | | |
| Beef: | | | | | | | | | |
| Eye of round, lean only, roasted | 3 oz | 85 | 156 | 53 | 5.9 | 2.4 | 2.7 | 0.2 | 56 |
| Ground beef, cooked, well done | 3 oz | 85 | 244 | 141 | 15.6 | 7.6 | 8.5 | 0.7 | 88 |

| Food item | Common Measure | Weight | Food energy | Energy from fat | Total fat | Fatty acids: Saturated | Fatty acids: Monounsaturated | Fatty acids: Polyunsaturated | Cholesterol |
|---|---|---|---|---|---|---|---|---|---|
| | | g | kcal | kcal | g | g | g | g | mg |
| Rib roast, lean and fat, roasted | 3 oz | 85 | 330 | 254 | 28.2 | 11.7 | 13.6 | 1.0 | 70 |
| Pork: | | | | | | | | | |
| Bacon, fried crisp | 2 slices | 13 | 73 | 56 | 6.2 | 2.2 | 3.0 | 0.7 | 11 |
| Ham, roasted | 3 oz | 85 | 187 | 85 | 9.4 | 3.2 | 4.2 | 1.1 | 80 |
| Lamb, loin chop: | | | | | | | | | |
| Lean only, broiled | 3 oz | 85 | 184 | 75 | 8.3 | 3.0 | 3.6 | 0.5 | 81 |
| Lean and fat, broiled | 3 oz | 85 | 269 | 177 | 19.6 | 8.4 | 8.2 | 1.4 | 85 |
| Veal cutlet, pan fried | 3 oz | 85 | 178 | 62 | 6.9 | 2.6 | 2.6 | 0.5 | 89 |
| Poultry, chicken, roasted: | | | | | | | | | |
| Dark meat, with skin | 3 oz | 85 | 215 | 121 | 13.4 | 3.7 | 5.3 | 3.0 | 77 |
| Dark meat, without skin | 3 oz | 85 | 174 | 75 | 8.3 | 2.3 | 3.0 | 1.9 | 79 |
| Light meat, with skin | 3 oz | 85 | 189 | 87 | 9.2 | 2.6 | 3.6 | 2.0 | 71 |
| Light meat, without skin | 3 oz | 85 | 147 | 34 | 3.8 | 1.1 | 1.3 | 0.8 | 72 |
| Related products: | | | | | | | | | |
| Beef liver, fried | 3 oz | 85 | 195 | 81 | 9.0 | 2.5 | 3.6 | 1.3 | 372 |
| Bologna (beef and pork) | 1 slice | 28 | 89 | 72 | 8.0 | 3.0 | 3.8 | 0.7 | 16 |
| Braunschweiger | 1 slice | 28 | 102 | 82 | 9.1 | 3.1 | 4.2 | 1.1 | 44 |
| Frankfurters (beef) | 1 frank | 57 | 184 | 152 | 16.8 | 6.8 | 8.2 | 0.7 | 27 |
| Salami, cooked (beef and pork) | 1 slice | 28 | 71 | 51 | 5.7 | 2.3 | 2.6 | 0.6 | 18 |
| **Miscellaneous (having ingredients of animal origin as sources of cholesterol)** | | | | | | | | | |
| Beef Pot pie | 1 piece | 210 | 515 | 275 | 30.5 | 7.9 | 12.9 | 7.4 | 42 |
| Beef stew | 1 cup | 245 | 220 | 95 | 10.5 | 4.4 | 4.5 | 0.5 | 72 |
| Cakes: | | | | | | | | | |
| Pound[3] | 1 slice | 33 | 160 | 88 | 10.0 | 5.9 | 3.0 | 0.6 | 61 |
| White, 2-layer, with chocolate icing[4] | 1 piece | 71 | 250 | 68 | 7.7 | 3.0 | 2.9 | 1.3 | 3 |
| Yellow, 2-layer, with chocolate icing[3] | 1 piece | 69 | 235 | 70 | 7.9 | 3.0 | 3.0 | 1.4 | 26 |
| Candy, milk chocolate | 1 oz | 28 | 145 | 80 | 9.0 | 5.4 | 3.0 | 0.3 | 5 |
| Chicken pot pie | 1 piece | 232 | 545 | 282 | 31.3 | 10.3 | 15.5 | 6.6 | 56 |
| Chicken a la king | 1 cup | 245 | 470 | 320 | 35.5 | 12.9 | 13.4 | 6.2 | 220 |
| Chili with beef | 1 cup | 253 | 254 | 75 | 8.3 | 3.4 | 3.4 | 0.5 | 133 |
| Cookies: | | | | | | | | | |
| Brownies, with chocolate icing[3] | 1 brownie | 25 | 105 | 47 | 5.3 | 2.0 | 2.3 | 0.7 | 8 |
| Chocolate-chip[5] | 4 cookies | 40 | 205 | 105 | 12.0 | 3.5 | 4.6 | 3.2 | 17 |
| Vanilla wafers[5] | 10 cookies | 40 | 185 | 59 | 6.7 | 1.7 | 2.8 | 1.7 | 20 |
| Crackers: | | | | | | | | | |
| Graham | 2 crackers | 14 | 55 | 11 | 1.3 | 0.3 | 0.5 | 0.4 | 0 |
| Saltines[6] | 4 crackers | 11 | 50 | 9 | 1.0 | 0.4 | 0.4 | 0.2 | 3 |
| Cupcakes, with chocolate icing[3] | 1 cupcake | 36 | 130 | 41 | 4.6 | 2.0 | 1.7 | 0.7 | 10 |
| Doughnuts, cake type[5] | 1 doughnut | 25 | 100 | 42 | 4.7 | 1.2 | 1.2 | 2.0 | 8 |
| Doughnuts, yeast-leavened[5] | 1 doughnut | 50 | 205 | 118 | 13.4 | 3.3 | 5.8 | 3.5 | 10 |
| Pizza with cheese[8] | 1 slice | 49 | 109 | 23 | 2.5 | 1.2 | 0.8 | 0.4 | 7 |
| Potatoes, french-fried (fried in edible tallow)[9] | 10 strips | 50 | 156 | 72 | 8.0 | 3.7 | 3.5 | 0.4 | 9 |

[1]Tr=Trace.
[2]Average of available data.
[3]Major sources of cholesterol are eggs and butter.
[4]Major sources of cholesterol are milk and butter.
[5]Major source of cholesterol is eggs.
[6]Major source of cholesterol is animal shortening.
[7]Source of cholesterol is milk solids.
[8]Source of cholesterol is cheese.
[9]Source of cholesterol is tallow.
U.S. Department of Agriculture Provisional Table. Revised Sept. 1988

# APPENDIX E

For additional information on Good Fats and Oils please contact:

Bronson Pharmaceuticals
1945 Craig Rd. P.O. Box 46903
St. Louis, Missouri 63146
1-800-235-3200
(mail order nutritionals, physician's newsletter)

Carlson Laboratories
15 College Drive
Arlington Heights, Ill. 60004
1-800-323-4141
(Retail stores, literature)

Solgar Vitamin and Herb Company
500 Willow Tree Road
Leonia, New Jersey 07605
1-800-645-2246
(Retail stores, literature)

Loriva Supreme Foods, Inc.
40-10 Oser Avenue
Hauppauge, New York 11788
1-800-94-LORIVA
(for culinary oils and recipes)

International Health Products
450 Commack Road
Deer Park, New York 11729
1-800-668-3556
(supplements)

# GLOSSARY

**acetylcholine:** a chemical transmitter for nerve impulses.

**adipose:** scientific name for body fat or fatty tissue.

**alpha-linolenic acid:** one of the two essential fatty acids that we cannot make and must obtain from food. It is extremely sensitive to oxygen, light, and high temperatures. Deficiency is linked to degenerative diseases.

**amino acid:** the building block of proteins; over 20 different amino acids are found in nature.

**antioxidants:** natural or synthetic substances (including some vitamins and minerals) that help inhibit destructive oxygen- and free radical-induced deterioration (oxidation) of fatty acids and other body components.

**arteriosclerosis:** a variety of conditions in which the artery walls thicken and lose their elasticity. Commonly referred to as "hardening of the arteries."

**atherogenic:** anything that has the ability to encourage the development of atherosclerosis.

**atherosclerosis:** a form of arteriosclerosis. The depositing of fatty plaques along the inner artery wall, thus narrowing the channel and reducing blood supply to vital organs.

**bile:** a fluid produced by the liver and stored in the gallbladder.

When the gallbladder contracts, the bile and its salts are secreted into the intestines to emulsify (break up) fats during digestion.

**cell membrane:** a double layer of fatty material (phospholipids) and proteins that surround cells in the body.

**cholesterol:** a fatty substance either made in our body or contained in foods of animal origin. It has important functions, but can be deposited in the blood vessels under unfavorable conditions.

**choline:** a member of the B vitamin family involved in nerve function and metabolism of fats. Lecithin is a good source as it contains phosphatidyl choline. Choline is used to make the neurotransmitter, acetylcholine.

**chylomicron:** a transporter for fat and cholesterol, made in our intestines that helps get digested food fats into the bloodstream where these fats can be distributed to our cells.

**cold pressed:** a commonly misused term which implies that an oil has been extracted without the use of chemical solvents.

**eicosapentaenoic acid (EPA):** a fatty acid abundant in cold-water fish and marine animals. It is the substance from which the body makes the series 3 prostaglandins. Its presence in the diet is associated with a reduced risk of arthritis, hypertension and cancer.

**emulsify:** to break up into smaller drops (of fat) by detergent action.

**essential fatty acid (EFA):** either of two fatty acids (linoleic and alpha-linolenic) that the body needs and cannot make from other substances.

**evening primrose:** a plant whose seeds contain the essential linoleic acid.

**fat:** in common usage, refers to substances that are hard at room temperature because they contain mostly saturated fatty acids.

**fatty acid:** a chemical structure of carbon and hydrogen with an organic acid group at one end. Fatty acids are building blocks of phospholipids, are used to make hormones and are fuel for our bodies.

**flax:** an ancient plant with seeds that are a rich source of alpha-linolenic acid, an essential fatty acid.

**free radicals:** unstable molecules that damage other molecules in the body's cells. Some of this cell damage is believed to lead to heart disease and cancer.

**gamma-linolenic acid (GLA):** a compound made from the essential fatty acid, linoleic acid, also found in hemp, borage, and evening primrose oils and mother's milk.

**high-density lipoprotein (HDL):** a carrier of fats and cholesterol that returns excess cholesterol from cells to the liver. Also called the "good" cholesterol.

**hydrogenation:** a commercial process by which liquid oils are turned into hard fats (margarines and shortenings) by a chemical process. Trans fatty acids created by this process can increase cholesterol levels.

**hypertension:** high blood pressure.

**lecithin:** a nutritional substance containing fatty acids, glycerol, a phosphate group and choline. Soybeans and egg yolks are good sources of lecithin. The substance is part of the structure of cell membranes and other cellular components.

**linoleic acid (LA):** One of the two essential fatty acids that we must obtain from our diet. The body makes several other important substances from it.

**lipid:** the scientific name for fats, oils, cholesterol, and other fatty substances.

**lipogenesis:** the formation and storage of fats in our body.

**lipolysis:** process by which fat cells release fat when you need it.

**lipoprotein:** fatty substances (fats, oils, cholesterol) are carried in this vehicle made of protein and phospholipids. Lipoproteins are transporters of lipids between our intestine, liver, and body cells. They are characterized by weight: VLDL-very low density; LDL-low density; HDL-high density; VHDL-very high density.

**low-density lipoprotein (LDL):** a transporter of fats and cholesterol in the bloodstream. Also termed, "bad" cholesterol, although new evidence indicates that the only "bad" cholesterol is cholesterol that is unprotected by antioxidants.

**molecule:** two or more atoms held together by a chemical bond.

**monounsaturated fatty acid (MUFA):** a fatty acid containing one double bond between carbon atoms somewhere in its fatty chain. MUFAs are considered to be healthy additions to the diet.

**neurotransmitter:** a chemical that serves as a communication link between neurons (brain cells).

**oil:** a liquid fat.

**oleic acid (OA):** a monounsaturated fatty acid found in olive, peanut, canola, pecan, macadamia and other oils.

**omega:** refers to the chemical structure found at the end of a fatty acid.

**omega 6:** a family of related fatty acids essential for human health.

**omega 3:** a family of related fatty acids essential to human health.

**partially hydrogenated:** an oil that has been chemically altered to produce a semi-solid fat. Many chemical changes take place in the fatty acid molecules during this process.

**phospholipid:** a class of fatty compounds found in cell membranes. Lecithin is the best-known example.

**plaque:** a deposit of fatty substances in the intima of the artery wall seen in atherosclerosis; also called atheroma.

**polyunsaturated fatty acid (PUFA):** a fatty acid that contains more than one double bond between carbon atoms in its chain. PUFAs include both natural, health-enhancing as well as unnatural, health-destroying kinds.

**prostaglandin (PG):** a fatty acid with hormone-like functions in the regulation of cell activity. Over 30 different prostaglandins are known. PGs are made from linoleic acid and linolenic acid and have wide reaching effects on the body, including contraction of smooth muscle and dilation of blood vessels.

**saturated fatty acid:** a fatty acid with no double bonds in the carbon chain. This arrangement makes it more solid and, in some cases, more dangerous to your health.

**steatorrhea:** an abnormal excess of fat in the stool.

**triglyceride (TG):** a molecule of fat or oil, the form in which fatty acids are stored in fat tissues and in the seeds of plants.

**ubiquinone:** a fat-soluble compound involved in the production of energy from carbohydrates. Also called co-enzyme Q10.

**unsaturated fatty acid (UFA):** a fatty acid with one or more double bonds between carbons in its chain. These fats are believed to be less dangerous to your health.

# INDEX

# ABOUT THE AUTHORS

The Nutrition Superbooks are based on material previously published in Keats Publishing's Good Health Guide series and in its newspaper *Health News & Review* (now *Health News Naturally*). Here are brief biographical sketches of the contributors to this volume.

**Richard A. Passwater, Ph.D.** is one of the most called upon authorities for information relating to preventive health care. A noted biochemist, he is credited with popularizing the term *supernutrition,* largely as a result of having written two bestsellers on the subject—*Supernutrition: Megavitamin Revolution* and *Supernutrition for Healthy Hearts.* His other books include *Easy No-Flab Diet, Cancer Prevention and Nutritional Therapies, Selenium as Food and Medicine, Trace Elements, Hair Analysis and Nutrition* (with Elmer M. Cranton, M.D.).

**Jeffrey Bland, Ph.D.** is CEO of HealthComm International, Inc., a leading global health communications firm, located in Gig Harbor, Washington. Before founding HealthComm, Dr. Bland was for 13 years a professor of chemistry at the University of Puget Sound in Tacoma, Washington. He is a former Senior Research Scientist at the Linus Pauling Institute of Science and Medicine and former director of a large medical laboratory in Washington State. Dr. Bland lectures widely on health and nutrition and has written and edited numerous books and articles for the scientific and popular press, including several works in the Good Health Guide series and the second of Keats Publishing's annual survey series, *A Year in Nutritional Medicine.*

**Jean Barilla** (editor and author) is a medical writer, lecturer and health consultant with degrees in Biology from New York University. She completed two years of medical school as part of a graduate program in biochemistry and has taught vitamin metabolism to medical students. Her writing appears in medical journals, medical-legal textbooks, magazines and newspapers. She writes and edits educational materials for physicians, health care personnel and the general public. Jean writes and edits a newsletter for physicians who use nutritional therapies in their practices and is the host of "Entertaining Health" a radio talk show in Fairfield County, Connecticut.

**Ingeborg M. Johnston** was born in Berlin, Germany, received her Certified Nutritionist diploma from the National Institute of Nutritional Education in 1985. She studied at the University of Berlin and the School of Nursing in Vienna, Austria and became a Registered Nurse in 1943. From 1980–1986 Ms. Johnston had a nutritional counseling practice in Pompano Beach, Florida.

**James R. Johnston** is the author of numerous articles on nutrition in professional journals and magazines. He received his Ph.D. from Occidental University in 1977. Since 1980, he has designed and authored courses and study guides for the National Institute of Nutritional Education (NINE), which graduates Certified Nutritionists.

**Beatrice Trum Hunter** is one of America's foremost food experts and consumer advocates, and a recipient of the prestigious Jonathan Forman Award of the Society for Clinical Ecology. She has written fourteen books in addition to two booklets in the Good Health Guide series. In terms of the kitchen, her *Whole Grain Baking Sampler* and *The Natural Foods Cookbook* have become standard equipment for natural foods cooks, with the latter selling well over two million copies. Ms. Hunter is food editor of *Consumers' Research Magazine*, lectures widely, and participates in workshops on many college campuses, as well as appearing on local radio and national television. Her books include: *The Sugar Trap and How to Avoid it*, and *The Great Nutrition Robbery.*

**Betty Kamen, Ph.D.** is coauthor, with Lynn Fraley, Ph.D., of *Nutrition in Nursing: The New Approach* and, with her husband, Si Kamen, of *Total Nutrition During Pregnancy, Kids Are What They Eat* and many other works on health and nutrition. She and Si Kamen have produced nationally recognized health-related TV shows and filmstrips.